O A P L

OXFORD AMERICAN PAIN LIBRARY

Menstrual Migraine

O A P L

OXFORD AMERICAN PAIN LIBRARY

Menstrual Migraine

Edited by

Susan Hutchinson, MD

Director and Founder, Headache Center
Orange County Migraine & Headache Center
UC-Irvine Medical Center
Irvine, CA

B. Lee Peterlin, DO

Director, Drexel University College of Medicine Headache Clinic
Assistant Professor, Department of Neurology
Drexel University College of Medicine
Philadelphia, PA

Executive Series Editor

Russell K. Portenoy, MD

Chairman of Pain Medicine & Palliative Care
Beth Israel Medical Center
New York, NY

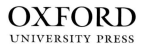

OXFORD
UNIVERSITY PRESS

2008

OXFORD
UNIVERSITY PRESS

Oxford University Press, Inc., publishes works that further
Oxford University's objective of excellence
in research, scholarship, and education.

Oxford   New York
Auckland   Cape Town   Dar es Salaam   Hong Kong   Karachi
Kuala Lumpur   Madrid   Melbourne   Mexico City   Nairobi
New Delhi   Shanghai   Taipei   Toronto

With offices in
Argentina   Austria   Brazil   Chile   Czech Republic   France   Greece
Guatemala   Hungary   Italy   Japan   Poland   Portugal   Singapore
South Korea   Switzerland   Thailand   Turkey   Ukraine   Vietnam

Copyright © 2008 by Oxford University Press, Inc.

Published by Oxford University Press, Inc.
198 Madison Avenue, New York, New York 10016

www.oup.com

Oxford is a registered trademark of Oxford University Press

Library of Congress Cataloging-in-Publication Data

Menstrual migraine / edited by Susan Hutchinson, B. Lee Peterlin.
p. ; cm. — (Oxford American pain library)
Includes bibliographical references.
ISBN-13: 978-0-19-536804-8 (standard ed. : alk. paper)
1. Menstrual cycle.   2. Migraine.
[DNLM: 1. Menstrual Cycle.   2. Migraine Disorders—etiology.   3. Menstruation.   4. Migraine
Disorders—complications.   5. Migraine Disorders—drug therapy.   6. Premenstrual Syndrome—
complications. WL 344 M548 2008] I. Hutchinson, Susan, 1956–   II. Peterlin, B. Lee.   III. Series.
RG161.M475 2008
618.1'72—dc22   2007042684

9 8 7 6 5 4 3 2 1
Printed in China
on acid-free paper

Acknowledgments

We would like to personally thank the outstanding authors for their excellent and significant contributions to this handbook. Special thanks also go to the hard-working efforts and constant encouragement of Yvonne Honigsberg and Tracy O'Hara of Oxford University Press. Finally, we thank you, the reader, for taking the time to learn more about this common and disabling condition. Together, we can help improve the quality of life of millions of women in this country who suffer from menstrually related migraine.

Contributors

Heather D. Adkins, MD
Nashville Neuroscience Group, P.C.
Nashville, TN

Sheena K. Aurora, MD
Co-director, Swedish Headache
Center
Seattle, WA

Jan Lewis Brandes, MD
Assistant Clinical Professor, Neurology
Vanderbilt University School of
Medicine
Nashville, TN

Dawn Buse, PhD
Director of Psychology, Montefiore
Headache Center
Assistant Professor, Department
of Neurology
Albert Einstein College of Medicine
New York, NY

Joan Golub, MD
Clinicol Instructor,
OB/GYN and Reproductive
Endocrinology
Brigham and Women's Hospital
Boston, MA

Susan Hutchinson, MD
Director and Founder, Headache
Center
Orange County Migraine & Headache
Center
UC-Irvine Medical Center
Irvine, CA

E. Anne Macgregor, MD
Director of Clinical Research
The City of London Migraine Clinic
London, UK

Stephanie Nahas, MD
Instructor of Neurology, Jefferson
Headache Center
Jefferson Medical School
Philadelphia, PA

B. Lee Peterlin, DO
Director, Drexel University College
of Medicine Headache Clinic
Assistant Professor, Department
of Neurology
Drexel University College of Medi-
cine
Philadelphia, PA

Ann I. Scher, PhD
Uniformed Services University of the
Health Sciences
Department of Preventive Medicine
and Biometrics
Bethesda, MD

Contents

Chapter 1

Introduction

Susan Hutchinson and B. Lee Peterlin

Menstrual migraine is a highly prevalent condition, affecting more than 50% of female migraine patients. This represents approximately 12 million women annually. Menstrual migraine is often reported to be more severe and longer in duration than nonmenstrual migraine. Unfortunately, it continues to be under-recognized and undertreated. Many women suffer with what they call their "period headache"; in other cases, headache is considered part of the premenstrual syndrome (PMS). Significant disability is associated with menstrual migraine and affects the ability to work, do household chores, and participate in social activities. As a result, the disability caused by menstrual migraine affects the family and the work environment; ultimately, many more than 12 million individuals are affected by menstrual migraine.

There are two types of menstrual migraine recognized by the International Headache Society: pure menstrual migraine (PMM) and menstrually related migraine (MRM) (Headache Classification Subcommittee of the International Headache Society, 2004).

Pure menstrual migraine is defined as migraine without aura, occurring exclusively on days −2 through 3+ during at least two of three menstrual cycles. Day 1 is defined as the onset of menstrual flow; there is no day "0." Pure menstrual migraine represents about 14% of female migraine patients. Menstrually related migraine is defined as migraine without aura, occurring on both days −2 through 3+ during at least two of three menstrual cycles and at other times of the month, and it affects about 46% of female migraine patients (Mannix and Calhoun, 2004). The term *menstrual migraine* will be used in this handbook to include both types, unless otherwise stated.

This handbook is meant to meet the needs of all those taking care of female patients to more effectively recognize and treat menstrual migraine. Many good articles and chapters have been published on menstrual migraine, but these articles are scattered among headache and primary care journals; they often focus on a particular aspect of menstrual migraine, and they are not easily accessible to everyone.

This handbook provides a very practical approach to menstrual migraine and is tailored to meet the needs of the busy primary care provider involved in treating the female patient, including physicians, nurse practitioners, and physician assistants in primary care specialties such as family practice, internal medicine, and OB-GYN. Neurologists, psychiatrists, and psychologists/therapists may also find this handbook useful. The authors of the chapters in this handbook have been carefully selected and represent some of the top experts in this field. Every attempt has been made to make this handbook the authoritative source on menstrual migraine for the busy primary care provider.

The book begins with a look at the epidemiology of menstrual migraine, which is followed by an in-depth look at the pathophysiology of menstrual migraine. We then move to practical tips and information on diagnosing menstrual migraine. A look at common comorbidities of the menstrual migraine patient is the theme of the next chapter. The next three chapters are among the most practical you may find on treatment recommendations for the menstrual migraine patient. A pharmacotherapy chapter covering acute, mini-preventive, and daily preventive approaches is followed by an enlightening chapter covering the controversial topic of estrogen use in these patients. Finally, the nonpharmacological treatment approaches, often very useful but overlooked by providers and patients, are covered and well described. Each chapter easily stands alone and can be used as a reference and learning tool for the busy provider who wants to focus on a particular aspect of menstrual migraine.

References

Headache Classification Subcommittee of the International Headache Society. (2004). The international classification of headache disorders: 2nd edition. *Cephalalgia*, **24(Suppl 1)**, 9–160.

Mannix LK, Calhoun AH, Calhoun AH. (2004). Menstrual migraine. *Current Treatment Options in Neurology*, **6**, 489.

Chapter 2

The epidemiology of migraine and the influence of sex hormones

B. Lee Peterlin and Ann I. Scher

Migraine is a common, chronic neurovascular disorder that presents with recurrent attacks that are often disabling. Risk factors for migraine include those that are associated with migraine per se (e.g., disease risk factors) and those that are associated with individual attacks or attack frequency (e.g., triggers). Hormonal changes throughout the life cycle and during the menstrual cycle appear both to influence pain proneness and to act as an attack trigger. For some women, attacks are more frequent—or are exclusively experienced—during specific times of the menstrual cycle (Silberstein and Merriam, 1999). Pure menstrual migraine (PMM) is defined as attacks of migraine without aura that occur "exclusively on day 1±2 (i.e., days −2 to +3) of menstruation in at least two out of three menstrual cycles and at no other times of the cycle." Menstrually related migraine (MRM) is defined as migraine without aura that occurs "day 1±2 (i.e., days −2 to +3) of menstruation in at least two out of three menstrual cycles and additionally at other times of the cycle." MRM and PMM have been recognized in the International Classification of Headache Disorders, second edition, at least partly as a result of recent epidemiologic research (Headache Classification Subcommittee of the International Headache Society [IHS], 2004).

In this chapter, we review the epidemiology of migraine, the impact of migraine, and the epidemiology of hormones and migraine, including MRM and PMM.

General migraine epidemiology

Incidence and prevalence

Epidemiological studies have greatly advanced our knowledge about migraine and have significantly impacted therapeutic recommendations for patients. Often, epidemiological studies focus on the *incidence* or *prevalence* of a disease in a specific population over a defined time period. Incidence is the rate of *new* cases of a disease in the at-risk population within a defined time period, while prevalence refers to the number of cases of a disease, both new and previously identified, that are present in a particular population at a given time. Most epidemiological studies of migraine measure 1-year prevalence, which is the proportion of the population meeting diagnostic criteria for migraine *and* who have had at least one attack in the last year. Some studies measure lifetime prevalence, which is the proportion of the population meeting diagnostic criteria for migraine, without the requirement of current or recent attacks. We first review the incidence and prevalence of migraine and then review the personal and societal impact that migraine may entail.

Incidence

In the general population, data suggest that the incidence of migraine occurs earlier in males than in females and that the incidence of migraine with aura occurs earlier than the incidence of migraine without aura. In males, the incidence of migraine with aura has been shown to peak at 5 years of age (at 6.6/1000 person-years), while migraine without aura peaks at 10 to 11 years (at 10/1000 person-years) (Stewart et al., 1991). In females, migraine with aura peaks at 12 to 13 years (at 14.1/1000 person-years), while migraine without aura peaks at 14 to 17 years (at 18.9/1000 person-years) (Stewart et al., 1991) (Fig. 2.1). Similarly, Breslau et al. (1991) showed that for any type of migraine, the mean age of migraine onset was almost 4 years earlier in boys than in girls. As the incidence of migraine peaks later in girls than in boys, the female-to-male preponderance that is seen in adult migraineurs is not evident in childhood; migraine in childhood is equally prevalent in girls and boys until approximately adolescence.

A recent study suggests that this pattern of increasing pain proneness after adolescence, at least in girls, may not be specific to migraine. LeResche and colleagues (2005) studied the relationship between pubertal development and the prevalence of four chronic pain conditions (headache, facial pain, back pain, and stomach pain) in 11- to 17-year-old adolescents identified from a managed care organization. Pubertal development was assessed using the Pubertal Development Scale (Petersen et al., 1988). Results showed that—for both boys and girls—pubertal development predicted the development of pain conditions better than age. In girls, pubertal development was positively associated with all four measured pain conditions (Fig. 2.2). For boys, pubertal development was positively associated with facial pain and back pain and was negatively associated with stomach pain.

Prevalence

It has been estimated that 12% of adults and 5% to 10% of children in the general population are affected by migraine in western hemispheric countries (Scher et al., 1999; Lipton et al., 2007; Stovner et al., 2007) (Fig. 2.3). In the United States alone, migraine affects approximately 28 million people. This in turn is reflected in the primary care setting, where migraine has been shown to be more prevalent than asthma, hypertension, and diabetes (Bensen and

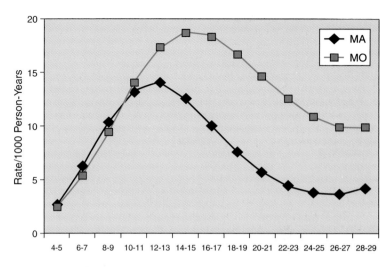

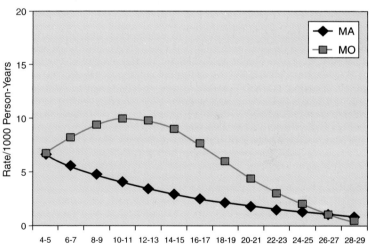

Figure 2.1 (*A*) Incidence of migraine with aura (MA) and migraine without aura (MO) in women. (*B*) Incidence of migraine with aura (MA) and migraine without aura (MO) in men. Adapted from Stewart et al., 1991.

Marano, 1998; Lipton et al., 2007). Migraine is most prevalent in mid-life between the ages of 25 and 55—the ages of greatest productivity for most adults (Scher et al., 1999; Stovner et al., 2007). It should be noted that, while attacks often remit after the age of 50 or so, migraine is not rare in late middle-age or in the elderly. For example, in the American Migraine Study (AIM) II, about 20%

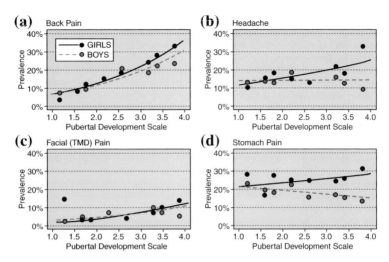

Figure 2.2 The relationship between pubertal development and the incidence of four pain conditions. Reprinted with permission, LeResche et al., 2005.

of women in their 50s and 8% of women in their 60s or older were found to have had a migraine attack within the past year. (The corresponding figures for men were 7% and 3% [Lipton et al., 2001b]). These and other results (Scher et al., 1999; Stovner et al., 2007) suggest that the 1-year prevalence of migraine decreases by about half after the 60s and that migraine is two to three times as prevalent in older women as in older men.

Migraine impact

According to the disease disability classes used in the World Health Organization Global Burden of Disease Study, using a person-trade-off method, severe migraine ("bedridden with severe pain") is more disabling than blindness, unipolar major depression, and paraplegia; and migraine is in the same disability class as active psychosis, dementia, and quadriplegia (Menken et al., 2000). In studies evaluating migraine disease burden, 67% of migraineurs reported that household work productivity was reduced by at least 50%, while 59% reported missing at least one family or social activity in the previous 3 months due to headache. In addition, 51% reported that work or school productivity was reduced by at least 50% during migraine attacks, 31% missed at least 1 day of work or school because of migraine in the 3 months prior to the survey, and 32% avoided making plans for fear of cancellations due to headaches (Lipton et al., 2001b; Brandes, 2002). This is supported by a recent population study showing that approximately 75% of migraineurs have a reduced ability to function and that 50% report severe impairment or require bed rest during acute attacks (Lipton et al., 2007).

Unfortunately, the diagnosis and treatment rates of migraine remain low, despite the recognition of the significant social, clinical, and economic impact of

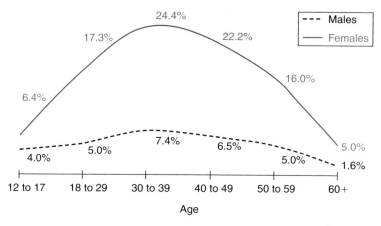

Figure 2.3 The 1-year period prevalence of migraine by age and sex. Reprinted with permission, Lipton et al., 2007.

migraine. In the AMS II, only 48% of subjects who met IHS criteria for a diagnosis of migraine had ever been diagnosed by a physician, and less than 50% of sufferers used prescription medications, half of whom (23%) combined it with over-the-counter pain relievers (Lipton et al., 2001b). In another general population study, of the 39% of headache sufferers who were candidates for preventative therapy or should be considered for preventative therapy, only 12.4% were currently using a preventative agent (Lipton et al., 2007).

Epidemiology of hormones and headache

Menarche, pregnancy, and menopause are hormonal milestones that are associated with major changes in the levels of cycling sex hormones. However, it is not just major hormonal changes that can affect headache disorders. The routine, cyclical hormonal changes that occur throughout a woman's normal menstrual cycle are often an important migraine trigger and may significantly affect the course of migraine in women (Peterlin and Loder, 2006).

A limited number of women of reproductive age report migraine attacks that occur only between the first 2 days before menses onset and the 3 days after menses onset, and at no other time of the menstrual cycle (i.e., PMM). However, many women report having migraine attacks that are triggered by menses and also occur at other times of their cycle outside of the perimenstrual period (i.e., MRM) (Headache Classification Subcommittee of the IHS, 2004).

Some of the first data linking sex hormones and migraine came from epidemiological studies. General population studies have shown that women are about three times more likely than men (17% versus 6%) to suffer from migraine

(Stewart et al., 1991; Lipton et al., 2007) (see Fig. 2.1). However, prior to puberty, migraine prevalence is roughly equal in boys and girls. It is not until adolescence that migraine prevalence and incidence become greater in girls than in boys. It has been estimated that 33% of women who develop MRM experience the onset of MRM at menarche (Epstein et al., 1975). After adolescence, migraine prevalence remains greater in women than in men for the rest of the life span—including after menopause (Scher et al., 1999; Stovner et al., 2007).

General population studies specifically assessing the prevalence and incidence of PMM and MRM are limited. One study by Courtier et al. (2003) evaluated a representative Dutch population sample of 1181 women. More than half (58%) of the women with regular cycles reported menstrual complaints, and 14% of these women reported migraine to be a frequent menstrual complaint. Thus 8% of Dutch women in the general population were shown to suffer from MRM, and approximately 1% from PMM.

In clinic-based studies of premenopausal migraineurs, MRM has been shown to occur in 17% to 50% of women, while PMM has been shown to occur in 5% to 8%. Thus, considering that the prevalence of migraine in women is approximately 17% in occidental countries, it can be estimated that 3% to 10% of women in the general population of Western-hemisphere countries suffer from MRM and 1% from PMM, numbers that closely match those found in the Dutch general population study of MRM and PMM (Silberstein and Merriam, 1999; Couturier et al., 2003; Lipton et al., 2007).

The increased incidence of migraine attacks in the perimenstrual period appears to be limited to attacks of migraine without aura (MO). Stewart et al. (2000) studied 81 women over a 98-day period and evaluated a total of 7219 headache diary days. They showed an excess risk of headache for MO (but not for migraine with aura) on days 1 and 2 of the menstrual cycle, as well as in the 2 days before onset of menses (Fig. 2.4). This is similar to a general population study by Russell et al. (1996), who evaluated the clinical characteristics of MO and migraine with aura (MA) and found that menstruation was a precipitating factor in MO but not likely in MA.

Similar to the study by Stewart et al. (2000), MacGregor and Hackshaw (2004) found an increased risk of headache in the 2 days before menstruation as well as during the first 3 days of menstruation. They conducted a diary study evaluating 155 women and analyzed a total of 693 menstrual cycles. During the 2 days before menstruation, women were 71% more likely to have migraine, with a relative risk of 1.71. During the first day of menstruation or during the preceding or following 2 days (i.e., day 1 of menses ±2 days), the chance of migraine was almost threefold greater than at all other times of the cycle, with a relative risk of 2.5. In addition, women were more than 3 times as likely to have a severe migraine on the first day of menstruation or during the preceding or following 2 days, with a relative risk of 3.41, and women were also almost 5 times more likely to experience vomiting in association with their migraines on or during days 1 to 3 of menstruation, with a relative risk of 4.69 (Holmes et al., 2001).

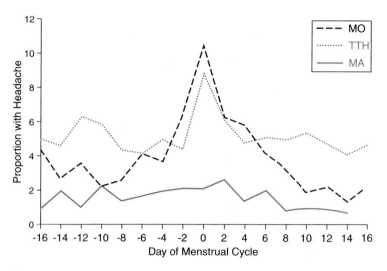

Figure 2.4 Headache prevalence by day of the menstrual cycle. MO: migraine without aura; TTH: tension-type headache; MA: migraine with aura. Adapted from Stewart et al., 2000.

MRM studies assessing the relationship between migraines and menstruation further emphasize the importance of recognizing and properly treating MRM. Several studies suggest that migraine attacks in the perimenstrual period are more severe, longer lasting, and less responsive to treatment compared with attacks outside the perimenstrual period. Stewart et al. (2000) showed that pain intensity was found to be greater for migraine headaches during the first 2 days of menstruation, although migraine duration was greater in the 3- to 7-day period before the onset of menses. However, Couturier et al. (2003) found that women with MRM reported that their MRM attacks were not just more severe but also of longer duration and more treatment resistant than nonmenstrually related attacks. Two other studies showed similar findings and are reviewed next.

Granella et al. (2004) evaluated the severity and responsiveness of MRM attacks to treatment compared with nonmenstrual migraine attacks in 64 women in a 2-month diary study. They found that migraine attacks in the perimenstrual period were significantly longer in duration, associated with greater work-related disability, and less responsive to treatment than those in the nonmenstrually related period. Specifically, whereas acute attack treatment with nonsteroidal anti-inflammatory drugs (NSAIDs) or triptans achieved pain freedom at 2 hours in 32.9% of nonmenstrually associated migraineurs, only 13.5% of women with MRM attacks achieved pain freedom at 2 hours with acute attack treatment. In addition, sustained pain freedom was attained in only 5.4% of MRM attacks compared with 24.2% of the nonmenstrually associated attacks. A recent study by Dowson et al. (2005) supports these finding and similarly showed that perimenstrual migraine attacks were significantly more severe, more disabling, and associated with a greater productivity loss compared with attacks outside this period.

Conclusion

Although epidemiological data have provided many insights into the relationship between menses and migraine, the exact cause of MRM remains unknown. Nonetheless, the existing epidemiological studies underscore the import in appropriately diagnosing MRM. It is now recognized that menstruation is a common migraine trigger for women and that MRM is associated with a significant disability, even greater than in nonmenstrually related migraine. Thus it is essential to recognize MRM. With an appropriate diagnosis, treatment can be tailored to the individual MRM sufferer's needs, and the most appropriate and best available care can be provided.

References

Bensen V, Marano M. (1998). Current estimates from the National Health Interview Survey, 1995. *Vital Heath Statistics*, **10:** 1–428.

Brandes JL. (2002). Global trends in migraine care: Results from the MAZE survey. *CNS Drugs*, **16(Suppl 1):** S13–S18.

Breslau N, Davis GC, Andreski P. (1991). Migraine, psychiatric disorders, and suicide attempts: An epidemiologic study of young adults. *Psychiatry Research*, **37:** 11–23.

Couturier EGM, Bomhof MAM, Neven AK, van Duijn NP. (2003). Menstrual migraine in a representative Dutch population sample: Prevalence, disability and treatment. *Cephalalgia*, **23:** 302–308.

Dowson AJ, Kilminster SG, Salt R, Clark M, Bundy MJ. (2005). Disability associated with headaches occurring inside and outside the menstrual period in those with migraine: A general practice study. *Headache: The Journal of Head and Face Pain*, **45:** 274–282.

Epstein MT, Hockaday JM, Hockaday TDR. (1975). Migraine and reproductive hormones throughout the menstrual cycle. *The Lancet*, **1:** 543–548.

Granella F, Sances G, Allais G, et al. (2004). Characteristics of menstrual and nonmenstrual attacks in women with menstrually related migraine referred to headache centres. *Cephalalgia*, **24:** 707–716.

Headache Classification Subcommittee of the International Headache Society. (2004). The international classification of headache disorders: 2nd edition. *Cephalalgia*, **24(Suppl 1):** 9–160.

Holmes WF, MacGregor EA, Dodick D. (2001). Migraine-related disability: Impact and implications for sufferers' lives and clinical issues. *Neurology*, **56(6 Suppl 1):** S13–S19.

LeResche L, Mancl LA, Drangsholt MT, Saunders K, Korff MV. (2005). Relationship of pain and symptoms to pubertal development in adolescents. *Pain*, **118:** 201–209.

Lipton RB, Bigal ME, Diamond M, Freitag F, Reed ML, Stewart WF. (2007). Migraine prevalence, disease burden, and the need for preventive therapy. *Neurology*, **68:** 343–349.

Lipton RB, Diamond S, Reed M, Diamond ML, Stewart WF. (2001a). Migraine diagnosis and treatment: Results from the American Migraine Study II. *Headache*, **7:** 638–645.

Lipton RB, Stewart WF, Diamond S, Diamond ML, Reed ML. (2001b). Prevalence and burden of migraine in the United States: Data from the American Migraine Study II. *Headache*, **41:** 646–657.

MacGregor EA, Hackshaw A. (2004). Prevalence of migraine on each day of the natural menstrual cycle. *Neurology*, **63:** 351–353.

Menken M, Munsat TL, Toole JF. (2000). The Global Burden of Disease Study: Implications for neurology. *Archives of Neurology*, **57:** 418–420.

Peterlin BL, Loder EW. (2006). Premenstrual headache: Diagnostic and pathophysiologic considerations. *Current Headache Reports*, **5:** 193–199.

Petersen AC, Crockett L, Richards M, Boxer A. (1988). A self-report measure of pubertal status: Reliability, validity, and initial norms. *Journal of Youth and Adolescents*, **17:** 117–133.

Russell MB, Rasmussen BK, Fenger K, Olesen J. (1996). Migraine without aura and migraine with aura are distinct clinical entities: A study of four hundred and eighty-four male and female migraineurs from the general population. *Cephalalgia*, **16:** 239–245.

Scher AI, Stewart WF, Lipton RB. (1999). Migraine and headache: A meta-analytic approach. In: Crombie IK (ed.), *The epidemiology of pain*. Seattle: International Association for the Study of Pain (IASP) Press, pp. 159–170.

Silberstein S, Merriam G. (1999). Sex hormones and headache 1999 (menstrual migraine). *Neurology*, **53(4 Suppl 1):** S3–S13.

Stewart WF, Linet MS, Celentano DD, Van NM, Ziegler D. (1991). Age- and sex-specific incidence rates of migraine with and without visual aura. *American Journal of Epidemiology*, **134:** 1111–1120.

Stewart WF, Lipton RB, Chee E, Sawyer J, Silberstein SD. (2000). Menstrual cycle and headache in a population sample of migraineurs. *Neurology*, **55:** 1517–1523.

Stovner L, Hagen K, Jensen R, et al. (2007). The global burden of headache: A documentation of headache prevalence and disability worldwide. *Cephalalgia*, **27:** 193–210.

Chapter 3

Migraine pathophysiology: Past to present

Sheena K. Aurora

Migraine is a common, often disabling neurovascular disorder. Although the full pathophysiology of migraine is not fully known, current theories suggest that it involves cortical spreading depression (CSD), neurogenic inflammation, and vasodilation. However, prior to the development of our current concepts of migraine, the pendulum of migraine pathophysiology swung between primary vascular or primary neural mechanisms. Harold G. Wolff, a pioneer of the vascular theory of migraine, proposed that the neurological symptoms of the migraine aura were caused by cerebral vasoconstriction and the headache by vasodilatation (Wolff, 1963). In 1941, the American neuropsychologist Karl S. Lashley provided the first piece of evidence that a neural mechanism for migraine with aura existed, by mapping the spread of his own visual scotoma and calculating that it spread at approximately 3 mm per minute (Lashley, 1941). Lashley's experience led to the concept of CSD, which 3 years later the Brazilian Aristides Leao would demonstrate in a rabbit model. Thus Lashley's (1941) and Leao's (1944) work would promulgate the neural theory of migraine. Newer imaging techniques have recently made it possible to study the very early events of migraine; thus both the primary vascular and primary neural theories have been reconciled by contemporary proponents of a neurovascular mechanism of the migraine attack.

There is an increasing body of evidence for the concept of central neuronal hyperexcitability as a pivotal physiological disturbance predisposing to migraine (Welch et al., 1990). The reasons for increased neuronal excitability are likely multifactorial, with an underlying genetic basis. Genetic studies have revealed an abnormality of calcium channels that has been introduced as a potential mechanism of interictal neuronal excitability (Ophoff et al., 1996). Mutant voltage-gated P/Q-type calcium channel genes likely influence excitatory or inhibitory presynaptic neurotransmitter release. It could therefore be hypothesized that genetic abnormalities result in a lowered threshold of response to a variety of triggers.

In the next sections, we first review the current concepts of the mechanisms of migraine aura and of head pain, and then discuss how they may be linked.

Mechanisms of aura

Because migraine is an episodic disorder that involves head pain and cortical phenomena that are not associated with structural abnormalities, investigations aimed at studying *how* the brain functions provide insight into migraine pathophysiology. The unpredictable and elusive nature of migraine has prevented many investigators from being able to systematically study migraine with aura (MA). However, with the advent of several functional MRI (fMRI) imaging techniques, including fMRI blood-oxygen-level-dependent imaging (fMRI-BOLD), perfusion-weighted imaging (PWI), and magnetoencephalography (MEG), this has changed. And recent studies using functional imaging of MA have made significant inroads into the current understanding of migraine.

Cao et al. (1999) were the first to be able to surmount the unpredictable occurrence of MA and measure the immediate-to-early events of the migraine attack. As migraineurs are known to be sensitive to linear stimuli, Cao's team used a red and green checkerboard for visual stimulation of migraine attacks. This technique reliably allowed for successful visual triggering of migraine attacks in 50% of subjects. Using the recently developed fMRI-BOLD technique, the authors were able to measure the second-to-second activation of the occipital cortex to visual stimulation in subjects who developed migraine. None of the 6 normal control subjects developed a headache, and they displayed normal patterns of BOLD signals on visual activation. However, 6 patients with MA and 2 patients with migraine without aura (MO) experienced visually triggered headache; 2 also had accompanying visual changes. Headache was preceded by suppression of initial activation that slowly propagated into contiguous occipital cortex regions at a rate ranging from 3 to 6 mm/min—similar to the rate Lashley calculated more than 65 years earlier. In addition, this neuronal suppression was accompanied by an increase in baseline contrast intensity indicative of vasodilatation and tissue hyperoxygenation. The baseline contrast increases that indicated tissue hyperoxygenation were similar to those witnessed in experimental CSD (Leao, 1944; Cao et al., 1999). These spreading events accompanied visually triggered headache whether or not it was associated with visual changes. Because patients were selected based on a history of visually triggered headache, generalizing these findings to all migraine patients must be done with caution. However, this study did help to clarify two significant points. First, it provided scientific evidence supporting the hypothesized mechanisms of CSD in migraine; second, it did *not* support the previously controversial findings of ischemia accompanying migraine aura.

As with fMRI, PWI is a relatively novel functional neuroimaging technique. PWI is particularly suited to short-lived events such as migraine aura. In a recent study using PWI, 28 spontaneous migraine attacks occurring in 19 different patients were studied (Sanchez del Rio et al., 1999). No significant changes in blood flow were observed in any of the MO attacks. However, during MA attacks, there was a relative reduction of cerebral blood flow in the occipital cortex contralateral to the visual defect and not in other brain regions. In addition, the hemodynamic changes that were seen were demonstrated only on PWI and not on diffusion-weighted imaging (DWI). Because DWI is sensitive to ischemia, this further supports the notion that MA is not an ischemic event.

MEG is also a functional imaging technique. It is used to measure the magnetic fields produced by electrical activity in the brain, similar to an electroencephalogram (EEG). In animals, the CSD's band of hyperexcited neurons traveling into sulci or fissures elicits an MEG signal. Barkley et al. (1990) studied MEG signals in humans. Using a seven-channel MEG, Barkley et al. reported direct current (DC) shifts in spontaneous migraine. Using the visual-trigger model developed by Cao et al., Bowyer et al. (1999) were also able to detect DC shifts when headache or aura was precipitated while using whole-head MEG, allowing more precise localization of signals than the seven-channel MEG. In Bowyer et al.'s study, headache was triggered in 5 of 8 migraine patients and none of 6 control subjects. DC-MEG shifts were observed in migraine subjects during visually triggered aura and in a patient studied during the first few minutes of spontaneous aura. No DC-MEG shifts were seen in control subjects. Large-scale MEG studies of patients undergoing spontaneous migraine attacks have not been possible because of the unpredictable nature of migraine and time of capture of these spontaneous events. However, both Cao et al. (1999) and Bowyer et al. (1999) provided additional evidence supporting the primary neural basis of migraine.

To date, CSD has yet to be successfully recorded in humans. However, although none of the above functional imaging studies directly demonstrate CSD, taken together, they do favor the neural basis of migraine.

Influence of hormones on cortical spreading depression

Migraine is 3 times more prevalent in women than in men. At least in part, the sex hormone differences may explain the female predominance (Martin and Behbehani, 2006; Welch et al., 2006). Both progesterone and estrogen may affect neuronal excitability via the regulation of several neurotransmitters, including the excitatory neurotransmitter glutamate and the inhibitory neurotransmitter GABA. Specifically, estradiol has been shown to augment *N*-methyl-D-aspartate (NMDA)-mediated glutamate receptor activity as well as to decrease GABA synthesis. Thus, estrogen generally lowers firing thresholds and enhances neuronal resting-discharge rates in the brain. In contrast, progesterone exerts inhibitory effects by enhancing GABA-mediated chloride conductance (Martin and Behbehani, 2006).

Both estrogen and progesterone have also been shown to influence CSD. Application of both hormones enhanced the repetition rate as well as the amplitude of SD in neocortical slices treated with hypotonic artificial cerebrospinal fluid. β-estradiol and progesterone also dose-dependently increased the amplitude of

SD induced by KCl microinjection, and both hormones exhibited a pronounced, persisting, and significant enhancement of long-term potentiation of the field excitatory postsynaptic potential in the neocortical tissues (Sachs et al., 2007). A recently published study also supports this relationship, but its researchers found that estrogen lowered the threshold of CSD (Haerter et al., 2007).

The association of estrogen has been studied with regard not only to neuronal response but also to gene regulation. Welch et al. (2006) hypothesized that estrogen may influence gene expression of molecules that counteract triggering and propagation of CSD, and that migraine attacks might occur if these balancing effects were mismatched. To examine this, CSD was induced in mouse brain by applying KCl. Gene expression was examined 2 hours later using cDNA array and reverse transcriptase-polymerase chain reaction. Of the more than 1180 genes examined, those consistently regulated by CSD included atrial natriuretic peptide (ANP) (upregulated) and neuropeptide Y (NPY) (downregulated) (Choudhuri et al., 2002). To explore the influence of estrogen, female mice were ovariectomized and, 1 week later, injected intraperitoneally for 7 days with 10 ng 17β-estradiol, while ovariectomized control animals were injected with 0.2 mL sesame oil. The estrogen-regulated proteins involved in signal transduction are G proteins and nitric oxide. NPY and ANP expression was higher with low estrogen, thus strengthening the theory that during low estrogen state, the brain is more susceptible to CSD.

Mechanism of pain

The brainstem, specifically the trigeminovascular system, has been implicated as playing a large role during migraine attack in both experimental and clinical studies (Raskin et al., 1987). It is hypothesized that a sterile inflammatory response occurs due to the release of neuropeptides (i.e., calcitonin-gene-related peptide [CGRP], cytokines, neurokinin A, and substance P) (Moskowitz, 1984). The development of novel antimigraine drugs for the treatment of migraine has been based predominantly on these animal models. This mechanism is further strengthened by the discovery of binding sites for the $5HT_{1B/1D}$ agonists on brainstem structures (Goadsby and Gundlach, 1991; Longmore et al., 1997).

The first human study to show activation in the brainstem used positron emission tomography (PET) scans of subjects during spontaneous migraine. Because PET lacks sufficient resolution for exact anatomical localization, the activation was hypothesized to be in the regions of the dorsal raphe nuclei (DRN), periaqueductal gray (PAG), and locus coeruleus (LC) (Weiller et al., 1995). In addition, a recent isolated case report found that the red nucleus (RN) and substantia nigra (SN) were activated in a spontaneous migraine attack (Welch et al., 1998). The same group of authors also reported that the RN and SN are activated in subjects with visually triggered migraine (Cao et al., 2002). The RN and SN are best known for their functional roles in motor control. The RN, however, has also been associated with pain. Numerous animal studies have documented a response of RN neurons to a variety of sensory and noxious stimuli. In a PET study performed on normal volunteers during capsaicin-induced pain, ipsilateral activation of the RN was documented. It remains to be clarified whether or not the RN is involved in the pain pathways or in the motor response to pain.

The PAG has a great influence on the nociceptive pathways, with extensive networks from the thalamus, hypothalamus, and autonomic nervous system. The PAG was found to be abnormal both interictally and ictally. Interictally, the PAG was shown to have an increased nonheme content that increased with the chronicity of migraine (Welch et al., 2001). Ictally, PET studies showed that the PAG was hyperactive (Bahra et al., 2001). The ventrolateral subdivision of the PAG (vlPAG) is of particular importance to the trigeminal nociceptive modulation (Knight and Goadsby, 2001). A genetic link to the predisposition of hyperactivity in the nociceptive system in migraine was recently established (Knight et al., 2002). Using a microinjection of the P/Q channel blocker ω-agatoxin IVA into the vlPAG, facilitation was noted in the trigeminal nociceptive activity. This study demonstrated the influence of both the P/Q-type calcium channels and PAG in trigeminal pronociception.

The influence of estrogen on this trigeminal vascular system has been elucidated by recent elegant experiments demonstrating the influence of cycling ovarian steroids on the peptide neurotransmitter systems in the trigeminal ganglion. Marked increase in gene expression of NPY occurred during the expected fall in estrogen of the estrus phase. The protein levels were further linked to the hormone levels. Because no changes were seen in levels of CGRP, the authors suggested modulation of nociceptive or cerebrovascular responses by estrogen via NPY. Sudden changes of this vasoactive peptide precipitated by falling levels of estrogen may trigger these attacks (Berman et al., 2002). These results have been mirrored using cutaneous receptive fields where enhanced sensitization of the trigeminal system during the latter halves of proestrus and estrus, which represent stages of the rat estrus cycle during and immediately following an abrupt decline in ovarian hormones, were noted (Martin and Behbehani, 2007).

Link between aura, neurogenic inflammation, and pain

The mystery of how a brain event (e.g., CSD) starting in an insensate part of the brain evolves into a painful disorder was recently elucidated. Bolay et al. (2002) demonstrated increase in flow of the middle meningeal artery (MMA) after CSD, which was produced by trauma. To clarify the mechanisms underlying these events, the trigeminal nerve was transected and demonstrated lack of the delayed phase of increased blood flow in MMA. Further, the expression of c-fos, a surrogate marker of pain, was increased in lamina I and II in trigeminal nucleus caudalis. There was also plasma protein extravasation noted in the experiment, which was noted to be mediated by neurokinin I. This landmark study clearly demonstrated the link between head pain of migraine and CSD, the putative mechanism of aura.

One of the other important mediators of plasma protein extravasation may be nitric oxide (NO). During migraine, NO metabolites (e.g., nitrites/nitrates) and secondary messengers of NO (e.g., cGMP) have been demonstrated to be increased in platelets (Stepien and Chalimoniuk, 1998; Shipmomura et al., 1999).

Migraine may be induced in patients after a 4- to 6-hour delay following nitroglycerin infusion (Olesen et al., 1993). The underlying pathogenetic mechanism has been noted to be a delayed inflammatory response in the dura matter, with increased expression of inducible NO synthase and upregulation of the proinflammatory cytokines interleukin (IL)-1β and IL-6 (Reuter et al., 2001). In addition, a recent study suggests that NO can either increase or decrease the mechanical responsiveness of nociceptors and that the action of NO might depend on baseline neuronal excitability (Levy and Strassman, 2004). Interestingly, as no patients have ever developed aura after glyceryl trinitrite infusion, it may therefore be hypothesized that NO may be induced *after* CSD.

As with NO, the neurogenic inflammation in migraine has also been associated with increased levels of the proinflammatory nuclear transcription factor nuclear factor (NF)-κB and increased levels of the cytokines IL-1 and IL-6 (Sarchielli et al., 2006a, 2006b). Estrogen inhibits NF-κB, IL-1, and IL-6. Thus, as estrogen levels decline, disinhibition of several proinflammatory substances occurs, and a woman's risk of migraine increases. The modulation of NO, NF-κB, and cytokines by estrogen may in part explain why women are more vulnerable to migraine during the perimenstrual period.

Evidence of interictal disturbances: Transcranial magnetic stimulation of occipital cortex in migraine

Now that we have explored mechanisms of aura, neurogenic inflammation, and head pain, we will turn our attention to what makes the migraine brain prone to an event such as CSD and thus to migraine. One mechanism for evaluating the interictal disturbances of the brain in migraine is transcranial magnetic stimulation (TMS).

TMS results in the generation of phosphenes. A phosphene is a visual effect whose source is within the eye itself and that is characterized by the sensation of seeing light. Phosphenes may be caused by simple mechanical stimulation of the retina, such as when you rub your eyes and "see stars," or from electrical or magnetic stimulation of the retina or occipital cortex, as with TMS. Phosphene generation by TMS of the occipital cortex can be used to evaluate occipital cortex excitability in migraine. Thus the use of TMS is particularly relevant to migraine, because enhanced excitability of the occipital cortex may underlie spontaneous and visually triggered migraine aura (Welch et al., 1990).

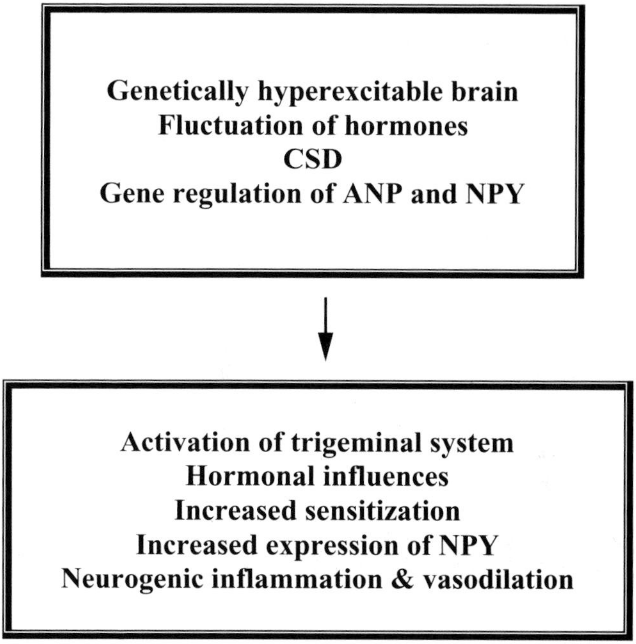

Figure 3.1. Migraine pathophysiology. CSD: cortical spreading depression; ANP: atrial natriuretic peptide; NPY: neuropeptide Y.

The first study using TMS in migraineurs reported a low threshold for generation of phosphenes in subjects with MA, inferring hyperexcitability of the occipital cortex (Aurora et al., 1999). In contrast, a second study inferred occipital cortex hypoexcitability in MA patients based on a lower prevalence of phosphenes stimulated by TMS in that study (Alfa et al., 1998). Important technical differences, such as the type of stimulator or coil size, might explain these conflicting findings (Aurora and Welch, 1999). Since these early reports, there have been two more studies on the occipital cortex using TMS, both confirming the initial reports of hyperexcitability (Aggugia et al., 1999; Aurora et al., 1999; Battelli et al., 2002). Although the effect of estrogen cycling has been examined using TMS, thus far no differences have been noted in phosphene generation in relationship to the menstrual period (Mulleners et al., 2001).

Conclusion

We currently conceive of a migraine attack as originating in the brain. Triggers of an attack initiate a depolarizing neuroelectric and metabolic event likened to the spreading depression described by Leao. This event activates the headache and associated features of the attack by mechanisms that remain to be determined but which appear to involve peripheral trigeminovascular and brainstem pathways. The excitability of cell membranes, which at least in part may be genetically determined, determines the brain's susceptibility to attacks. Factors that increase or decrease neuronal excitability modulate the threshold for triggering attacks. Hormonal fluctuations throughout a woman's life cycle, as well as in the routine menstrual cycle, can alter a woman's threshold for migraine. In particular, the estrogen withdrawal associated with the routine menstrual cycle in women is associated with a number of events that can make women particularly vulnerable to migraine.

References

Afra J, Mascia A, Gerard P, Maertens de Noordhout A, Schoenen J. (1998). Interictal cortical excitability in migraine: A study using transcranial magnetic stimulation of motor and visual cortices. *Annals of Neurology*, **44:** 209–215.

Aggugia M, Zibetti M, Febbraro A, Mutani R. (1999). Transcranial magnetic stimulation in migraine with aura: Further evidence of occipital cortex hyperexcitability. *Cephalalgia*, **19:** 465.

Aurora SK, Al-Sayed F, Welch KMA. (1999). The threshold for magnetophosphenes is lower in migraine. *Neurology*, **52:** A472.

Aurora SK, Cao Y, Bowyer SM, Welch KMA. (1999). The occipital cortex is hyperexcitable in migraine: Evidence from TMS, fMRI and MEG studies (Wolff Award 1999). *Headache*, **39:** 469–476.

Aurora SK, Welch KMA. (1999). Phosphene generation in migraine [Letter to the editor]. *Annals of Neurology*, **45:** 416.

Bahra A, Matharu MS, Buchel C, Frackowiak RSI, Goadsby PJ. (2001). Brainstem activation specific to migraine headache. *The Lancet*, **357:** 1016–1017.

Barkley GL, Tepley N, Nagel-Leiby S, Moran JE, Simkins RT, Welch KMA. (1990). Magnetoencephalographic studies of migraine. *Headache*, **30:** 428–434.

Battelli L, Black KR, Wray SH. (2002). Transcranial magnetic stimulation of visual area V5 in migraine. *Neurology*, **58:** 1066–1069.

Berman N, Puri V, Cui L, Klein R, Welch KMA. (2002). Trigeminal ganglion neuropeptide cycle with ovarian steroids in a model of menstrual migraine. *Headache*, **42:** 438.

Bolay M, Reuter U, Dunn A, Huang Z, Boas D, Moskowitz M. (2002). Intrinsic brain activity triggers trigeminal meningeal afferents in a migraine model. *Nature Medicine*, **8:** 136–142.

Bowyer SM, Aurora SK, Burdette DE, Moran JE, Tepley N, Welch KMA. (1999). *Neuromagnetic Measurements of Evoked and Spontaneous Migraine with Aura*. Presented at the Congress of the International Headache Society, June 1999, Barcelona, Spain.

Cao Y, Aurora SK, Vikingstad EM, Patel SC, Welch KMA. (2002). Functional MRI of the red nucleus and occipital cortex during visual stimulation of subjects with migraine. *Neurology*, **59:** 72–78.

Cao Y, Welch KM, Aurora S, Vikingstad EM. (1999). Functional MRI-BOLD of visually triggered headache in patient with migraine. *Archives of Neurology*, **56:** 548–554.

Choudhuri R, Cui L, Yong C, et al. (2002). Cortical spreading depression and gene regulation: Relevance to migraine. *Annals of Neurology*, **51:** 499–506.

Goadsby PJ, Gundlach AL. (1991). Localization of 3H-dihydroergotamine-binding sites in cat central nervous system: Relevance to migraine. *Annals of Neurology*, **29:** 91–94.

Haerter KE, Kudo C, Moskowitz MA. (2007). Cortical spreading depression and estrogen. *Headache*, **47:** S79–S85.

Knight YE, Barsch T, Kaube H, Goadsby PJ. (2002). P/Q-type calcium-channel blockade in the periaqueductal gray facilitates trigeminal nociception: A functional genetic link for migraine. *Journal of Neuroscience*, **22:** 1–6.

Knight YE, Goadsby PJ. (2001). The periaqueductal gray matter modulates trigeminovascular input: A role in migraine? *Neuroscience*, **106:** 793–800.

Lashley KS. (1941). Patterns of cerebral integration indicated by the scotoma of migraine. *Archives of Neurology and Psychiatry*, **46:** 331–339.

Leao AAP. (1944). Spreading depression of activity in the cerebral cortex. *Journal of Neurophysiology*, **8:** 379–390.

Levy D, Strassman A. (2004). Modulation of dural nociceptor mechanosensitivity by the nitric oxide-cyclic GMP signaling cascade. *Journal of Neurophysiology*, **92:** 766–772.

Longmore J, Shaw D, Smith D, et al. (1997). Differential distribution of 5-HT1D and 5-HT1B immunoreactivity within the human trigeminocerebrovascular system: Implications for the discovery of new anti-migraine drugs. *Cephalalgia*, **17:** 835–842.

Martin VT, Behbehani M. (2006). Ovarian hormones and migraine headache: Understanding mechanisms and pathogenesis—Part 1. *Headache*, **46:** 3–23.

Martin VT, Behbehani MM. (2007). Sensitization of the trigeminal sensory system during different stages of the rat estrous cycle: Implications for menstrual migraine. *Headache*, **47:** 552–563.

Moskowitz MA. (1984). The neurobiology of vascular head pain. *Annals of Neurology*, **15:** 157–168.

Mulleners WM, Chronicle EP, Koehler PJ, Vredeveld JW. (2001). Longitudinal assessment of cortical excitability in women with menstrual migraine. *Cephalalgia*, **21:** 392.

Olesen J, Iversen HK, Thomsen LL. (1993). Nitric oxide supersensitivity: A possible molecular mechanism of migraine pain. *Neuroreport*, **4:** 1027–1030.

Ophoff RA, Terwindt GM, Vergouwe MN, et al. (1996). Familial hemiplegic migraine and episodic ataxia type-2 are caused by mutation in the Ca^{+2} channel gene CACNL1A4. *Cell*, **87:** 543–552.

Raskin NH, Hosobuchi Y, Lamb S. (1987). Headache may arise from perturbation of the brain. *Headache*, **27:** 416–420.

Reuter U, Bolay H, Janen-Olsen I, et al. (2001). Delayed inflammation in rat meninges: Implications for migraine pathophysiology. *Brain*, **124:** 2490–2502.

Sachs M, Pape HC, Speckmann EJ, Gorji A. (2007). The effect of estrogen and progesterone on spreading depression in rat neocortical tissues. *Neurobiological Diseases*, **25:** 27–34.

Sanchez del Rio M, Bakker D, Wu O, et al. (1999). Perfusion weighted imaging during migraine spontaneous visual aura and headache. *Cephalalgia*, **19:** 701–707.

Sarchielli P, Alberti A, Baldi A, et al. (2006b). Proinflammatory cytokines, adhesion molecules, and lymphocyte integrin expression in the internal jugular blood of migraine patients without aura assessed ictally. *Headache*, **46:** 200–207.

Sarchielli P, Floridi A, Mancini ML, et al. (2006a). NF-kB activity and iNOS expression in monocytes from internal jugular blood of migraine without aura patients during attacks. *Cephalalgia*, **26:** 1071–1079.

Shipmomura T, Murakami M, Kotani K, Ikawa S, Kono S. (1999). Platelet nitric oxide metabolites in migraine. *Cephalalgia*, **19:** 218–222.

Stepien A, Chalimoniuk M. (1998). Level of nitric oxide-dependent cGMP in patients with migraine. *Cephalalgia*, **18:** 631–634.

Weiller C, May A, Limmroth V, et al. (1995). Brainstem activation in spontaneous human migraine attacks. *Nature Medicine*, **1:** 658–660.

Welch KMA, Brandes JL, Berman NEJ. (2006). Mismatch in how oestrogen modulates molecular and neuronal function may explain menstrual migraine. *Neurology and Science*, **27:** S190–S192.

Welch KMA, Cao Y, Aurora SK, Wiggins G, Vikingstad EM. (1998). MRI of the occipital cortex, red nucleus, and substantia nigra during visual aura of migraine. *Neurology*, **51:** 1465–1469.

Welch KMA, D'Andrea G, Tepley N, Barkley G, Ramadan NM. (1990). The concept of migraine as a state of central neuronal hyperexcitability. *Neurology Clinics*, **8:** 817–828.

Welch KMA, Nagesh V, Aurora SK, Gelman N. (2001). Periaqueductal grey matter dysfunction in migraine: Cause or the burden of illness? *Headache*, **41:** 629–637.

Wolff HG. (1963). *Headache and other head pain* (2nd ed.). New York: Oxford University Press.

Chapter 4

Tips and pearls for the diagnosis of migraine and menstrually related migraine

Stephanie Nahas and B. Lee Peterlin

Migraine is a highly prevalent neurovascular disorder often associated with significant disability. In the primary care setting, it has been shown to be more prevalent than hypertension, diabetes, and asthma (Martin, 2004) (Fig. 4.1). Although migraine is prevalent in both genders, it is three times more common in women, occurring in 17% of women and 6% of men in the general population (Lipton et al., 2007).

Hormonal influences, in part, may explain the female predominance. The major hormonal milestones (menarche, pregnancy, and menopause) are linked to shifts in cycling hormone levels and often have a significant impact on headache disorders. In addition, the rhythmic hormonal changes that occur throughout a woman's menstrual cycle affect headache disorders and may in fact have a more substantial effect over time, given their regular and generally predictable occurrence (Peterlin and Loder, 2006).

It has been estimated that menstrually related migraine (MRM) affects up to 60% of female migraineurs (Lay and Payne, 2007) and accounts for a significant proportion of the affliction's substantial economic burden to society (Ferrari, 1998). Unfortunately, large general population studies show that only 48% of patients with headache fulfilling criteria for migraine are ever given such a diagnosis, let alone that of MRM, by their health-care providers (Lipton et al., 2001).

Correct diagnosis is essential for recommending appropriate, effective treatment for headache disorders. This may be particularly challenging given the lack of strong biomarkers of disease, thus necessitating reliance on clinical features. In addition to lack of knowledge of the diagnostic criteria for headache disorders, other barriers to the successful treatment of MRM include incomplete history-taking (e.g., not inquiring if headaches occur in association with a woman's menstrual cycle), failure to recognize common contributors (e.g., medical and psychiatric comorbidities, caffeine and analgesic-medication overuse, disability), and failure to identify signs or symptoms that may point to a treatable or

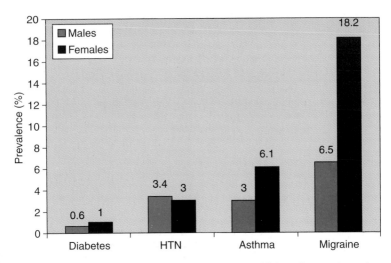

Figure 4.1 Prevalence of common diseases. The prevalence of diabetes, hypertension, and asthma are for those 45 years of age and younger. HTN, hypertension. Adapted with permission, Martin VT, 2004.

secondary cause of headache. All of these factors can impact both the headache diagnosis and treatment choices and, when not considered, can lead to incomplete or incorrect diagnoses and subsequent, suboptimal, ineffective, or inappropriate treatment. This chapter reviews how to achieve an accurate headache diagnosis, particularly with regard to MRM, using the following steps:

- Identify the important aspects of a focused headache interview.
- Utilize headache diaries/calendars. (This step is imperative!)
- Review the tools available to aid in assessing the impact of disability and common comorbidities associated with migraine.
- Recognize when special consideration is needed.

The headache history

A patient's history is arguably the most important factor in achieving a correct headache diagnosis. Eliciting this history accurately and efficiently, however, often poses a challenge to even the most experienced clinician. Using a systematic approach, guided by established diagnostic criteria for headache disorders and aimed at identifying contributors to the disorder, will help minimize frustration and maximize patient–physician rapport and satisfaction. The headache itself must first be classified based on the features of the pain itself and the associated symptoms (see later sections). Beyond this, it is also imperative to assess for sleep disturbances, depression, anxiety, abuse, post-traumatic stress disorder, weight problems, and the influence of medication and other substances. Affective and headache disorders not only are comorbid and may influence one another but also share many commonalities of treatment. Also, inadequate sleep, whether due to primary insomnia or a condition such as obstructive sleep apnea, negatively affects headaches, which may further impair sleep (Silberstein et al., 2007). Obesity is associated with risk of progression to chronic daily headache (Scher et al., 2003). Some medications and other substances may aggravate headache due to side effects, and, moreover, when acute headache medication or substances such as caffeine are overused, headaches typically worsen (Sheftell and Bigal, 2006).

Making a diagnosis of migraine and menstrually related migraine

To diagnose menstrual or menstrually related migraine, one must first understand the definition of migraine headache, how it differs from tension-type headache, and what makes a migraine "menstrually related." The diagnosis of migraine is made by applying the criteria set forth in the International Classification of Headache Disorders, second edition (ICHD-II) (Headache Classification Subcommittee of the International Headache Society, 2004). Migraine headaches are hours-long (between 4 and 72) attacks of characteristic head pain associated with typical nonpain symptoms. After establishing the duration of the headache attacks, "U-MAP" the pain:

- **U**nilateral
- **M**oderate to severe intensity
- **A**ggravation by or avoidance of physical exertion
- **P**ounding/pulsating/throbbing quality

Two or more of the above criteria are needed for migraine diagnosis. Next, at least one of the following two associated symptoms must be present:

1. Nausea and/or vomiting
2. Photophobia *and* phonophobia

If a single criterion of duration, pain, or associated symptoms is missing, the diagnosis is probable migraine. ("Probable migraine" is, in fact, a diagnosis; its name does not imply diagnostic uncertainty.)

In contrast to migraine, tension-type headaches are often described as "not migraine." (They are not unilateral, not moderate to severe in intensity, not aggravated by activity, not pounding in character, etc.) However, one or two "migraine" features may be permissible for the diagnosis of tension-type headache, and vice versa. Thus, many patients believe their migraines are merely tension-type headaches, because they may be bilateral or may not cause total incapacity. When the criteria are applied, many patients have both migraine and tension-type

Table 4.1 Headache triggers and aggravating factors

Category	Evidence exists	Anecdotal
Foods, beverages, and substances	Alcohol, caffeine, nitroglycerine, carbon monoxide	Fasting, nitrates, MSG, chocolate, nuts, cheese, aspartame, sucralose, amines, citrus, banana, vegetables, dairy, fatty fried food, wheat, seafood
Physical	Strenuous exercise, forceful coughing or chewing, sexual intercourse	
Stress	Home, work, interpersonal	
Environment	Sunlight, weather shifts	Altitude, seasonal allergens
Sleep		Too much, not enough, disturbed cycle
Hormonal	Menses	Pregnancy, menopause, BCP

BCP: birth control pill. *Source:* Krymchantowski and Soraya, 1999; Zivadinov et al., 2003; Bigal and Krymchantowski; 2006; Patel et al., 2006; Wöber et al., 2006.

headaches. This may affect treatment decisions, which again underscores the importance of an accurate diagnosis.

MRM occurs within the context of an episodic migraine disorder, wherein attacks happen consistently in association with the menstrual cycle (occurring within 2 days of onset of menses to 3 days after the onset of menses), as well as at other times of the month. In contrast, pure menstrual migraine (PMM) occurs exclusively in concert with menses. MRM attacks tend to be more severe, disabling, and difficult to treat than non-MRM attacks (Johannes et al., 1995). Again, this emphasizes the need for rapid and accurate diagnosis to provide optimal therapeutic interventions.

Direct questions related to each criterion will establish the correct diagnosis. However, a simple three-question inventory serves as a moderately sensitive (81%) and specific (75%) screening tool with excellent positive predictive value (93%) for the presence of a migraine disorder (Lipton et al., 2004). This screener is particularly useful for the busy primary care provider or women's health specialist. Patients may fill out the questionnaire in the waiting room, prompting them to think more about a health problem that may have thus far gone unaddressed. It also opens the door to further discussion. In women, if a patient screens positive for migraine, it should prompt the clinician to ask whether her migraines occur in association with her menses. If a woman is unsure, or even if she feels certain, a headache calendar should be provided to document the co-occurrence of migraine with the menstrual cycle, as recall may be biased by stereotypic notions about menstrual symptoms and may influence the recounting of the history (Peterlin and Loder, 2006). A simple screening questionnaire in conjunction with a headache diary or calendar often leads to more specific and successful treatment, resulting in reduction or resolution of disability and enrichment of a woman's quality of life.

Importance of headache calendars

Headache calendars are invaluable tools for both physicians and patients. In addition to addressing the specific criteria of the ICHD-II for migraine, MRM, and PMM, it is important to elicit modifying factors, including precipitants or triggers, exacerbants, and relieving factors. Potential precipitants and exacerbants need to be recognized and avoided when possible, while relieving factors need to be identified and reinforced. This knowledge can be obtained rapidly and effectively from headache diaries. In addition, the knowledge gained from headache calendars may help guide the choice of other therapeutic options. For example, when migraines are identified to occur in association with a woman's menses, short-term prophylactic therapies starting 1 to 2 days before the expected onset of headache should be considered. As another example, when it is recognized that acute medication is being overused, posing an issue of safety or contributing to the perpetuation of recurrent headaches, nonpharmacological therapies or bridge therapy should be considered.

Headache diaries and calendars can be quite helpful in identifying these contributors, while at the same time serving the obvious purpose of establishing a more specific diagnosis, such as with MRM or medication overuse headache (MOH). In addition, headache diaries and calendars also function to confirm or establish attack frequency, response to treatment, and disability due to headache.

Patients need to be coached and reminded of the importance of an accurate record of headache, not only for diagnostic and therapeutic purposes but also for their own edification. Until a patient undertakes this sometimes tedious exercise, there are often misconceptions regarding the number of headache attacks in a given month, the reliability of triggers, and the amount of medication used. Moreover, when kept for months at a time, one has proof of whether interventions have made any difference. In a study of such record keeping, 72% of patients affirmed that communication with their physician was enhanced, and 70% indicated significant satisfaction with their medical care as a result. Among physicians, 91% agreed patient–physician communication became more effective, and all found diaries helpful in assessing disability across patients (Baos et al., 2005).

Ideally, a headache diary ought to contain all the activities undertaken that may have led to (or, even more important, that did not lead to) headache, and all activities missed due to headache, as a measure of disease burden. Similarly, all foods, environmental exposures, weather shifts, sleep changes, perceived stressors, medications taken (daily and as-needed medications, including over-the-counter preparations, taken for any purpose), and, of course, the onset of the menstrual cycle need to be tallied. The details of the headache attack, including the time of onset, duration, intensity, associated symptoms, and if/how relief was achieved that day, are essential. A headache calendar condenses this information to a single page, saving time for both patients and clinicians by illustrating patterns of headache occurrence and recurrence. These tools are invaluable in identifying quickly the relevant precipitants, aggravants, and relieving factors crucial to diagnosis and treatment.

Migraine triggers—facts and myths exposed

What are true migraine triggers? Many are perceived, but few are substantiated with scientific evidence (see Table 4.1) A recent prospective study using sophisticated statistical analyses of detailed diary data showed that the strongest and most consistent trigger is menstruation, increasing the hazard of occurrence or persistence of headache or migraine by up to 96% (Wober et al., 2007). Identification of menstruation as a trigger provides an easy-to-hit therapeutic target. Specific treatment options for MRM are discussed in detail in Chapters 6, 7, and 8.

In addition to menstruation, the Wober study identified other factors, such as stress, lack of exercise, low atmospheric pressure, sunshine for longer than 3 hours per day, and air advection from the polar regions, that also may increase the risk of migraine and serve as triggers. Tiredness and muscle tension also predict the occurrence of headache, although these may represent dopaminergic prodromal phenomena (Peroutka, 1997). Interestingly, this study showed reduced risk of headache with divorce, progesterone-only contraception, and consumption of beer. No influence was seen from chocolate, cheese, nuts, red wine, cigarette smoke, other odors, hunger, or sleep disturbances—all commonly perceived as headache triggers. It must, of course, be remembered that the absence of evidence is not the evidence of absence. In this study in particular, patients may have consciously avoided these potential precipitants, thus masking their contribution. Additionally, triggers can be highly specific to individuals.

What about chocolate, the oft-maligned treat shunned by many a migraineur? It has been suggested that biogenic amines in chocolate may provoke headache, that the caffeine in chocolate may play a role, or that eating chocolate prior to a headache may merely be a hypothalamically driven migraine prodromal craving (Scharff and Marcus, 1999). Moreover, a double-blind, controlled study showed that chocolate is no more likely to trigger migraine than carob (Marcus et al., 1997). Let them eat chocolate cake!

The multitude of potential triggers for migraine, real and perceived, should be discussed in detail with patients. Once a patient's true and false triggers are identified, patients can avoid precipitants whenever possible and may regain pleasure from formerly avoided circumstances or substances.

Assessment of disability: Helpful tools

Assessment of disability is essential. When it is significant, treatment must be more aggressive. The Migraine Disability Assessment (MIDAS) tool was developed to determine the impact of headache on a patient's daily living in terms of time lost from occupational or school duties, household maintenance, and non-work activities (Stewart et al., 1999). Patients enumerate the number of days lost completely in addition to those during which at least half the day was unproductive or unfulfilling. It has been validated, translated into many languages, and proved useful not only in assessing disability burden at a particular point in time but also as an outcome measure of the effect of headache treatment. In addition, it quantifies the total number of headache days and their average intensity, thus allowing a further sense of the overall impact of headaches for an individual.

The Headache Impact Test (HIT) is another effective and easy-to-use tool for assessment of headache-related disability. It measures the impact headaches have on a person's ability to function on the job, at home, at school, and in social situations. The HIT was developed by a team of headache experts in collaboration with the psychometricians who developed the SF-36 health assessment tool. A short form of 6 questions (HIT-6) was derived from an initial pool of 54 items. It takes approximately 2 minutes to complete, yielding an accurate description of the impact headaches are having on an individual's quality of life. The HIT has been validated and translated into dozens of languages and is used extensively in both clinical practice and for scientific purposes (Kosinski et al., 2003).

Who needs further consideration and investigation?

The presence of other medical illnesses may signify a potential secondary cause of headache or offer an additional target of therapy that may also benefit the headache disorder. In migraineurs who also have hypertension, a β-blocker such as timolol may be used; this also has proven efficacy in headache prevention (Silberstein and Young, 2006). Conversely, β-blockers may be contraindicated or less desirable in migraineurs with asthma or depression. Psychiatric conditions are particularly important to identify, as many are comorbid with migraine, especially depression (Couch et al., 1975). In addition, many antidepressants, such as the tricyclic antidepressants and serotonin-norepinephrine reuptake inhibitors, are also effective migraine-preventive agents. However, one must also determine whether a patient has bipolar disorder, as antidepressants without mood stabilizers could provoke a manic episode in such patients (Peterlin and Ward, 2005). Screening for depression may be done simply with a tool such as the Beck Depression Inventory, a 21-item questionnaire (Beck et al., 1996), or the Patient-Health Questionnaire module for depression (PHQ-9), a 9-item screener (Kroenke et al., 2001).

Making the connection between headache and such comorbidities may not always be straightforward, but it is crucial to diagnosis. It is essential to ask about or screen for such things, lest they be missed. In addition, these outside influences, or other signs and symptoms, may implicate a secondary cause for headache that requires further investigation. A simple mnemonic may aid in this process: SNOOP (Doddick, 2003). While more applicable to headache diagnosis in general, there is still a role for this approach in MRM/PMM, as even a headache with a readily identifiable trigger may have a morbid or easily treatable underpinning:

Systemic symptoms (fever, weight loss), secondary risks (HIV, known cancer)

These may indicate a serious underlying medical illness such as widespread infection, which could penetrate the central nervous system and lead to headache or, in the case of HIV, make one susceptible to central nervous system infection. Fortunately, evidence suggests most headaches are not caused or worsened by primary and metastatic brain tumors. In fact, headache is the presenting symptom in only up to 20% of cases, although headache does develop eventually in approximately 60%. Infratentorial tumors are more likely to cause headache in the occipital region; glioblastoma multiforme is often associated with dull pain, while meningioma is associated with throbbing pain; and migraineurs may be more susceptible to brain tumor headache (Schankin et al., 2007).

Neurological symptoms/signs (altered consciousness, focal deficits)

When present, intracranial pathology such as stroke must be ruled out. Stroke itself can be a migraine trigger (Nahas et al., 2007). It should also be remembered that benign variants of migraine with aura may present this way (Sarkari and Soni, 1974).

Onset—sudden or split-second

The so-called "thunderclap headache" often is benign, but several secondary causes need to be ruled out. The differential diagnosis includes subarachnoid hemorrhage, unruptured intracranial aneurysm, aneurysmal expansion or thrombosis, cervical arterial dissection, cerebral venous thrombosis, retroclival hematoma, pituitary apoplexy, stroke, reversible cerebral vasoconstriction syndrome, spontaneous cerebrospinal fluid leak, hypertensive crisis, intracranial infection, and colloid cyst of the third ventricle, as well as other, less common causes. Computed tomography, lumbar puncture, and magnetic resonance imaging (including arteriography and venography) will exclude or confirm these causes in the vast majority of cases (Schwedt et al., 2006).

Older—new or progressive headache over age 50

Migraine prevalence peaks in middle age, but incidence typically drops off after age 50 (Lipton et al., 2007). Temporal arteritis (Wykes and Cullen, 1985) and other arteridities (Ward and Levin, 2005) commonly present with new or progressive headache in the older individual (even a woman who is still menstruating) and may be indistinguishable from typical primary headaches. Often, but not always, constitutional and visual symptoms are present. Prompt recognition and treatment are vital in preventing permanent neurological sequelae, most notably blindness.

Prior history—first, newly progressive, or different headaches from the patient's usual headaches

Any unusual headache beyond what is described above deserves further investigation.

Conclusion

Any clinician may become skilled and comfortable with proper headache diagnosis. Essential to the task are knowledge of the ICHD-II criteria, a structured interview, knowledge of tools to aid in the assessment, and recognition of when further investigation is required. Only when the diagnosis is solid may treatment be effective and patients' lives be made better, or even saved. Practice, assessment, and reassessment are the keys to success.

References

Baos V, Ester F, Castellanos A, et al. (2005). Use of a structured migraine diary improves patient and physician communication about migraine disability and treatment outcomes. *International Journal of Clinical Practice*, **59:** 281–286.

Beck AT, Steer RA, Brown GK. (1996). *Manual for the Beck Depression Inventory* (2nd ed.). San Antonio, TX: Psychological Corp.

Couch JR, Ziegler DK, Hassanein RS. (1975). Evaluation of the relationship between migraine headache and depression. *Headache*, **15:** 41–50.

Dodick DW. (2003). Clinical clues and clinical rules: Primary vs secondary headache. *Advanced Studies in Medicine*, **3:** S550–S555.

Ferrari MD. (1998). The economic burden of migraine to society. *PharmacoEconomics*, **13:** 667–676.

Headache Classification Subcommittee of the International Headache Society. (2004). The international classification of headache disorders: 2nd edition. *Cephalalgia*, **24(Suppl 1):** 9–160.

Johannes CB, Linet MS, Stewart WF, Celentano DD, Lipton RB, Szklo M. (1995). Relationship of headache to phase of the menstrual cycle among young women: A daily diary study. *Neurology*, **45:** 1076–1082.

Kosinski M, Bayliss MS, Bjorner JB, et al. (2003). A six-item short-form survey for measuring headache impact: The HIT-6™. *Quality of Life Research*, **12:** 963–974.

Kroenke K, Spitzer RL, Williams JBW. (2001). The PHQ-9: Validity of a brief depression severity measure. *Journal of General Internal Medicine*, **16:** 606–613.

Lay CL, Payne R. (2007). Recognition and treatment of menstrual migraine. *Neurologist*, **13:** 197–204.

Lipton RB, Bigal ME, Diamond M, Freitag F, Reed ML, Stewart WF. (2007). Migraine prevalence, disease burden, and the need for preventive therapy. *Neurology*, **68:** 343–349.

Lipton RB, Diamond S, Reed M, Diamond ML, Stewart WF. (2001). Migraine diagnosis and treatment: Results from the American migraine study II. *Headache*, **41:** 638–645.

Lipton RB, Dodick D, Sadovsky R, Chessman AW. (2004). A 3 item screening instrument had moderate sensitivity and specificity for detecting migraine headaches. *Evidence-Based Medicine*, **9:** 56.

Marcus DA, Scharff L, Turk D, Gourley LM. (1997). A double-blind provocative study of chocolate as a trigger of headache. *Cephalalgia*, **17:** 855–862.

Martin VT. (2004). Simplifying the diagnosis of migraine headache. *Advanced Studies in Medicine*, **4:** 200–207, 209.

Nahas SJ, Pineda CC, Shaw JW, et al. *Headache in Acute Cerebrovascular Disease: A Prospective Study.* Presented at the American Academy of Neurology Annual Meeting, Boston, MA, April 2007.

Peroutka SJ. (1997). Dopamine and migraine. *Neurology*, **49:** 650–656.

Peterlin BL, Loder EW. (2006). Premenstrual headache: Diagnostic and pathophysiologic considerations. *Current Headache Reports*, **5:** 193–199

Peterlin BL, Ward TN. (2005). Neuropsychiatric aspects of migraine. *Current Psychiatry Reports*, **7:** 371–375.

Sarkari NB, Soni VK. (1974). Migraine variants with focal neurological manifestations. *The Journal of the Association of Physicians of India*, **22:** 907–913.

Schankin CJ, Ferrari U, Reinisch VM, Birnbaum T, Goldbrunner R, Straube A. (2007). Characteristics of brain tumour-associated headache. *Cephalalgia*, **27:** 904–911.

Scharff L, Marcus DA. (1999). The association between chocolate and migraine: A review. *Headache Quarterly*, **10:** 199–205.

Scher AI, Stewart WF, Ricci JA, Lipton RB. (2003). Factors associated with the onset and remission of chronic daily headache in a population-based study. *Pain*, **106:** 81–89.

Schwedt TJ, Matharu MS, Dodick DW. (2006). Thunderclap headache. *Lancet Neurology*, **5:** 621–631.

Sheftell FD, Bigal ME. (2006). Medication overuse headache. *CONTINUUM Lifelong Learning in Neurology*, **12:** 153–169.

Silberstein SD, Young WB. (2006). Preventive treatment. *CONTINUUM Lifelong Learning in Neurology*, **12:** 106–132.

Silberstein SD, Dodick D, Freitag F, et al. (2007). Pharmacological approaches to managing migraine and associated comorbidities—clinical considerations for monotherapy versus polytherapy. *Headache*, **47:** 585–599.

Stewart WF, Lipton RB, Whyte J, et al. (1999). An international study to assess reliability of the Migraine Disability Assessment (MIDAS) score. *Neurology*, **53:** 988–994.

Ward TN, Levin M. (2005). Headache in giant cell arteritis and other arteritides. *Neurological Sciences*, **26(Suppl 2):** S134–S137.

Wober C, Brannath W, Schmidt K, et al. (2007). Prospective analysis of factors related to migraine attacks: The PAMINA study. *Cephalalgia*, **27:** 304–314.

Wykes WN, Cullen JF. (1985). Headache and temporal arteritis. *Scottish Medical Journal*, **30:** 42.

Chapter 5

Comorbidities in migraine

Jan Lewis Brandes and Heather D. Adkins

Comorbidity is commonly used to refer to the greater than coincidental association of two conditions or disorders in the same individual. While the evidence for the comorbidity of depression and migraine has been well established, the term is sometimes used quite broadly to include numerous disorders, many of which have only recently been recognized as truly comorbid with migraine. The associations that in the past have not been clearly established are becoming so, as newer research reveals evidence for comorbidity and not merely coexistence.

Migraine and premenstrual syndrome

Premenstrual syndrome (PMS) is a cyclical mood disorder characterized by the presence of one or more affective (e.g., depression, irritability, anxiety, confusion, social withdrawal) or somatic (e.g., breast tenderness, abdominal bloating, swelling of extremities) symptoms during the 5 days before menses. PMS is also associated with relief of the above symptoms within 4 days after the onset of menstruation. Premenstrual dysphoric disorder (PMDD) is a more severe form of PMS. Patients with PMDD have five or more of the affective or physical symptoms mentioned, beginning during the last week of the luteal phase and remitting during the week after menses. The disturbance may interfere with work, school, or social activities and cannot be related to premenstrual exacerbation of another disorder such as depression (Peterlin and Loder, 2006). The estimated prevalence of PMS in women is 48% to 90%, whereas PMDD is about 10 times less frequent, occurring in about 5% to 8% of women.

Studies have suggested an association between migraine headaches and PMS. Facchinetti et al. (1993) reported that 64% of patients with pure menstrual migraine and 33% of those with menstrually related migraine met diagnostic criteria for PMS. The association of these disorders has raised the question of whether severity of the symptoms of PMS and menstrual migraine could be related. In other words, does the presence of one disorder potentiate the other? In the study by Facchinetti et al. (1993), a history of migraine headaches was not associated with increased frequency or severity of PMS symptoms when compared with women suffering from PMS who did not have a history of migraines. A study by Beckham et al. (1992) found the severity of PMS symptoms to be moderately correlated with the headache index during premenstrual and menstrual time intervals of the menstrual cycle. A small study by Martin and colleagues (2006) also suggested that the presence and severity of headache may relate to severity of PMS symptoms in female migraineurs. To date, no study has specifically examined the relationship between PMDD and migraine, although Martin's study suggests that an association is likely. Large, prospective studies are needed to investigate the possible relationship between headache severity and PMS symptoms, as these could have therapeutic implications for both disorders.

Depression and migraine

Migraines are known to cause significant lost productivity and decreased quality of life, with part of the morbidity being attributable to psychiatric symptomatology. More than 30% of migraineurs, compared with 10% of individuals without migraine, have a lifetime prevalence of major depression (Hamelsky and Lipton, 2006). The association between migraine and depression is the most widely recognized psychiatric comorbidity; however, migraine is also linked with generalized anxiety disorder, panic disorder, and bipolar disorder.

A number of studies have identified an association between migraine and increased prevalence of depression. In 1990, Merikangas et al. demonstrated an association between migraine and depression by interviewing 457 subjects to assess the presence of psychiatric syndromes and migraine headache. This was the first study to show a strong association between migraine and major depression in an unselected sample. In 2000, Breslau and colleagues demonstrated similar findings in a population-based study of persons between the ages of 25 and 55 years. Subsequent large-scale population studies have reported similar results, demonstrating that persons with migraine are 2.2 to 4.0 times more likely to have depression.

Several prospective, longitudinal studies suggest that there is a bidirectional relationship between migraine and depression. In 2003, Breslau et al. reported that in a population-based cohort studied over a 2-year period, having baseline depression increased the risk of incident migraine but not other severe headaches. This study also showed the risk of depression to be significantly higher in those with baseline migraine but not in patients with other types of severe headaches. This finding is consistent with results from prior studies by Breslau et al. (1994, 2000), which also demonstrated an interactive relationship between depression and migraine. In these studies, the relative risk of incident migraine in people with preexisting depression ranges from 2.8 to 3.5 times higher than that in individuals without depression. Similarly, the relative risk of new-onset depression in patients with preexisting migraine ranges from 2.4 to 3.8 times higher compared to those without migraine.

Findings of a bidirectional influence between migraine and major depression suggests the presence of a common neurobiologic substrate, with involvement of both monoamine (serotonin [5HT] and dopamine) and peptide neurotransmitters. Serotonin has been implicated in mood disorders, sleep disorders, migraine, and tension-type headache, with studies most strongly implicating $5HT_1$ receptor involvement. There is also emerging evidence linking dopamine dysregulation to migraine, considering that migraine prodrome is often characterized by dopaminergic symptoms, and antidopaminergic compounds are helpful in treatment. These data suggest that headache, somatic symptoms, and major depression may be linked through dysfunction of the serotonergic and dopaminergic systems. Establishing a common neurobiology of migraine and mood disturbance could influence therapeutic strategies directed at serotonin and dopaminergic systems.

Anxiety disorders have also been associated with migraine, with the relationship being demonstrated in both clinical and community-based studies (Facchinetti, Tarabusi, and Nappi, 1998). Whereas a bidirectional relationship has been suggested with migraine and depression, the onset of anxiety typically precedes the onset of migraine. In 2004, a cross-sectional study by McWilliams et al. showed a link between migraine and anxiety. In this study, 9.1% of persons with migraine, compared with 2.5% of those without migraine, had comorbid generalized anxiety disorder. Merikangas et al. (1990) also reported a strong association between migraine and anxiety disorders, with generalized anxiety disorder and social phobia exhibiting the strongest relationship. An association between migraine and panic disorder has also been reported. Studies have also addressed the co-occurrence of depression and anxiety. Merikangas and colleagues (1990) found a twofold increased risk of migraine among subjects with both major depression and anxiety disorder. A possible connection between bipolar disorder and migraine has not been studied extensively, but a strong association has been reported by McIntyre et al. (2006). In this study of approximately 37,000 respondents, there was a 34.7% incidence of migraine in women with bipolar disorder, compared with 14.7% of women without bipolar disorder.

The association of migraine with mood and anxiety disorders indicates the importance of screening patients presenting with any of these diagnoses for the presence of other comorbidities. This would be useful for directing treatment, considering that many medications for migraine can aid in treatment of psychiatric disorders, and vice versa.

Abuse and post-traumatic stress disorder

Both abuse and post-traumatic stress disorder (PTSD) have been shown to be associated with migraine (Peterlin et al., 2007a, 2007b; Tietjen, 2007). In addition, while migraine prevalence has long been established as higher in women, abuse is also reported to have a higher prevalence in women. (Breslau et al., 2003). The role of estrogen in migraine, at least in part, is thought to explain the higher prevalence of migraine in women (Brandes, 2006), and Seedat et al.

(2005) have suggested that the higher prevalence of PTSD may be attributable to the higher rates of sexual and physical abuse in women.

The lifetime prevalence of abuse in the general population is reported to be about 25%. The prevalence of abuse (physical, sexual, and emotional) ranges from 13% up to 27% in childhood, and a host of population-based studies show an association between abuse and headache.

Two recent clinic-based studies have shown that abuse may be associated with migraine (Peterlin et al., 2007a; Tietjen, 2007). In a retrospective study of 183 headache patients, Peterlin et al. (2007a) found that 40% of chronic daily headache sufferers, compared to 27.3% of episodic migraineurs, had a history of physical and/or sexual abuse. In addition, a large, prospective, clinic-based study by Tietjen (2007) found similar results. Of 1032 women, 92% of whom had migraine, physical or sexual abuse was reported in 38%, and approximately 12% reported both physical and sexual abuse in the past. Overlaps between maltreatment types were also noted (Tietjen, 2007).

In women with a history of childhood sexual maltreatment, 36% experienced physical abuse, 29% described fear for life, 52% witnessed abusive behaviors between adults as a child, and 45% reported drug/alcohol abuse by adults in their childhood home. Approximately one-fifth of patients ($n = 180$) reported childhood onset of sexual abuse, physical abuse, or fear for life. Interestingly, the author (Tietjen, 2007) found no differences in age or race between migraineurs but did find that women with a history of maltreatment had lower household income and lower education level than did women without a history of maltreatment. A higher proportion of women reporting physical abuse, sexual abuse, or fear for life related to abuse had chronic headache. Headache disability, depression, and somatic symptoms were also higher in patients reporting a history of maltreatment. History of maltreatment was significantly associated with severity of depression. Their findings concluded that childhood maltreatment was more common in women with migraine and depression than in those with migraine alone. They further identified that sexual abuse in childhood amplified the association with migraine and depression if the abuse occurred both before and after age 12. These authors offer their results as support of the hypothesis that stressful events, such as childhood maltreatment, may lead to a variety of conditions characterized by serotonin dysfunction, including migraine, depression, and anxiety. This work suggests that gently asking about maltreatment and the age at which it was or is being experienced should be considered in the evaluation of migraineurs with depression and more frequent headache.

A recent pilot study by Peterlin et al. (2007b) examined the frequency of PTSD in patients with episodic and chronic migraine using the PTSD checklist (civilian version). Although the relative frequency of depression was noted to be higher in chronic migraineurs (55.2%) than in episodics migraineurs (21.9%,) the relative frequency of PTSD was reported in a greater percentage of chronic migraineurs (42.9%) compared with episodic migraineurs (9.4%), even after adjusting for depression.

Migraine and irritable bowel syndrome

The association between migraine and gastrointestinal disorders is well recognized in epidemiological studies. Cole et al. (2006) examined 97,593 patients with irritable bowel syndrome (IBS) and showed that patients in the IBS group had a 60% higher risk of migraine compared with 27,402 control subjects.

Common pathophysiological mechanisms of IBS and migraine are likely related to the gut–brain axis. The enteric nervous system has numerous neurotransmitters that may serve as a plausible link between IBS and migraine. Serotonin is presumed the most likely involved neurotransmitter, considering its role as the primary neurotransmitter in the digestive tract and its known involvement in migraine.

Migraine and endometriosis

Among women of reproductive age, migraine and endometriosis are fairly common, with prevalence rates of about 15% to 20% and 10%, respectively. Both endometriosis and migraine have greater than coincidental associations with asthma, chronic fatigue syndrome, and fibromyalgia. The shared comorbidities among migraine and endometriosis raise the possibility that there may be an association between them.

Two studies provide evidence for such a relationship between migraine and endometriosis. In 2004, Ferrero et al. demonstrated an increased frequency of migraine headache in a population of women with endometriosis. In the study, 33.8% of the 133 patients with endometriosis suffered from migraine, compared with 15.1% in the control group. Tietjen and colleagues (2006) also reported an association between migraine and endometriosis, demonstrating that a cohort of 55 migraineurs had a higher frequency of menorrhagia and endometriosis. In a more recent study, Tietjen et al. (2007b) confirmed their previous findings, noting the presence of endometriosis in 22% of a sample of 171 women with migraine versus 9.6% for the control group. This study also evaluated characteristic of headaches in patients with endometriosis and found that migraineurs with endometriosis have more frequent and disabling headaches and an increased likelihood of associated affective and pain-related comorbidities.

Migraine and fibromyalgia

Fibromyalgia syndrome (FMS) is a chronic pain syndrome of unknown etiology characterized by diffuse pain for greater than 3 months and tenderness in specific sites. There is a well-documented association between headache and fibromyalgia in the literature. Headache is often reported in about 50% of fibromyalgia patients. Conversely, fibromyalgia has increased incidence in patients with migraine headache.

Marcus and colleagues, in 2005, supported prior studies by demonstrating increased prevalence of headache in patients with diagnosed fibromyalgia. They analyzed 100 treatment-seeking fibromyalgia patients and found a 76% incidence of headaches. Approximately 63% of these patients with headaches were diagnosed with migraine. In this study, headache predated fibromyalgia symptoms in 46% of the patients by an average of 7 years.

Studies of headache-patient populations have also supported the link between migraine and fibromyalgia. A study by Ifergane et al. (2005) demonstrated a 22% prevalence of fibromyalgia in 92 patients with episodic migraine, showing a much higher incidence than the 2% to 3% rate found in the general population.

The association between migraine and FMS has led to theories establishing a common pathophysiological mechanism. According to a recent review by Sarchielli and Filippo (2007), a growing body of evidence supports involvement of peripheral and central sensitization disturbances in both disorders, which is presumably due to increased glutamate transmission. If future studies support this finding, it could have implications for future therapies directed against glutamate receptors (e.g., NMDA receptors).

Obesity

Obesity has been shown to be associated with migraine. Several neurotransmitters and proteins that are associated with adiposity and/or feeding behavior have been linked with migraine, including serotonin, ghrelin, and orexin; others, such as adiponectin, have been suggested (Holland et al., 2005; Peterlin et al., 2007c). Here, we focus on the epidemiological studies suggesting an association between migraine and obesity.

Increasing body mass index as a risk factor for the development of chronic daily headache has been noted (Scher et al., 2003b) and has promoted an interest in the relationship between migraine and obesity, two highly prevalent conditions in the United States. The association between body mass index and migraine-attack frequency and severity was established in a population-based study by Bigal et al. (2006), but not with migraine prevalence. Given that obesity is strongly associated with disorders of mood, specifically depression and anxiety, in school-age children, adolescents, and women, and that the bidirectionality of migraine and depression has been shown in longitudinal studies (Breslau, 2003), Tietjen et al. (2007c) explored the effect of depression and anxiety on the migraine–obesity relationship. In their study of 721 migraine patients, both anxiety and depression were associated with obesity. Worsening attack severity and frequency were associated with increasing body mass index, but the association of obesity with migraine frequency was found to be significant only in migraineurs with depression. Obesity was also found to be associated with increased attack frequency in migraineurs with anxiety, but not after controlling for depression. The relationship between obesity, disability, and anxiety continued to be significant even when controlled for depression. The study did not have a control population, nor did the larger population-based study control for mood disorders; however, a previous study (Tietjen et al., 2007a) did show that major depression was strongly associated with both chronicity and with significant headache-related disability.

It has been suggested that both studies provide important insight with regard to the association with obesity. Both studies evaluated obesity using the body mass index, an estimate of *total body fat*. It is likely that obesity is indeed associated with migraine, although the association has not been entirely defined. Studies smaller than the general population studies evaluating the migraine–obesity association (yet still relatively large for clinic studies) have not able to show this association. However, as previously noted, the absence of evidence is not the evidence of absence. It may be that *regional* or *abdominal obesity*, as estimated by the waist-to-hip ratio, could be at least part of the explanation for why large, general population migraine studies have been able to capture the association using a nonregional estimate of obesity, and two smaller, yet still relatively large, clinic-based studies have not (B. L. Peterlin, personal communication). This may suggest that a more specific and/or sensitive estimate of obesity than body mass index may be needed, such as waist-to-hip ratio, and future research is needed to evaluate this potential.

Migraine and sleep disorders

Migraine attacks may be triggered by changes in sleep/wake patterns. Weekend migraine attacks have long been associated with oversleeping or longer sleep duration (Rains and Poceta, 2006). Sleep deprivation related to difficulty in achieving sleep onset and/or maintaining sleep is frequently reported in migraine and is more commonly reported as a trigger for migraine in women than in men, according to one study by Rasmussen (1993).

In a group of 1283 migraineurs (84% women), Kelman and Rains (2005) reported that more than half reported difficulty initiating and maintaining sleep at least occasionally. Based on reported sleep patterns, patients were assigned to groups of short, normal, or long sleep groups. In the short sleep group patients, who routinely slept 6 hours per night, more severe headache was reported, along with more sleep-related headache. Sleep disturbances, including more awakening headache and difficulty falling asleep or staying asleep, were more common in those with chronic migraine than in those with episodic migraine.

Calhoun et al. (2006) reported a higher prevalence of nonrestorative sleep in 147 women with chronic migraine. All patients denied feeling "refreshed" on awakening, and 83.7% reported feeling "tired" on awakening. Difficulty falling asleep was reported by two-thirds and sleep medications were being used by more than half of the women in the study. Seventy-three percent were overusing acute medications.

Calhoun and Ford's (2007) recent pilot study of 43 patients suggests that there is an important relationship between sleep and chronic daily headache. The study concluded that improvement in nonrestorative sleep and poor sleep habits may be an efficacious treatment method for transformed migraine. Patients who received cognitive-behavioral therapy for sleep experienced a statistically significant reduction in headache frequency and intensity vis-à-vis the placebo group. While only 25% of placebo patients reverted to episodic migraine, roughly half of the treated patients successfully reverted. Additionally, of the patients who adhered to all five of the behavioral sleep modification instructions, only one did not revert, whereas among those who were nonadherent to three or more instructions, none reverted.

Polysomnography in headache patients is limited to small studies, but in one such study of 25 headache clinic patients complaining of morning headache, sleep disorders were diagnosed in 13 of the 25 patients. Periodic limb movements of sleep, fibromyalgia, and obstructive sleep apnea were among the diagnoses made on the basis of formal polysomnography. In a slightly larger group of 288 patients, treatment of the primary sleep disorder, with the exception of periodic limb movements of sleep patients, was reported to resolve headache (Pavia et al., 1995, 1997). Snoring has been reported as a risk factor for the development of chronic headache in a population-based study by Scher et al. (2003a), who also noted that the association to snoring was independent of weight, gender, hypertension, age, or another sleep disorder.

Efforts should be made to instruct migraineurs in sleep hygiene and to encourage them to establish a regular sleep schedule throughout the entire week. Going to bed at the same time each evening and awakening at the same time may be adequate in some women for eliminating the role of sleep fluctuations as a migraine trigger. Particular attention to sleep may be needed during the menstrual cycle in women who have comorbid premenstrual syndrome as another source of sleep fragmentation. If behavioral measures are not successful, rapid-onset sleep medications may be offered and preventive migraine medications that promote or enhance sleep may be increased during the vulnerable period for sleep difficulties.

Migraine and ischemic vascular events

The relationship between migraine and stroke has been debated for a number of years. A recent meta-analysis by Etminan and colleagues (2005) including 11 retrospective case-control and three prospective studies demonstrated an increased risk of stroke in subjects with migraine. The pooled relative risk was 2.16, and the risk was similar for migraine with aura and migraine without aura. Since the publication of the meta-analysis, an additional, large-scale, prospective cohort study by Kurth et al. (2005) has demonstrated a 1.7-fold increased risk of ischemic stroke for women who reported migraine with aura. The risk was highest in women aged 45 to 55 years and was not seen in older women.

The Stroke Prevention in Young Women Study (Kurth et al., 2005) compared 386 women with first ischemic stroke with 614 age-matched control subjects. When compared with women without headache, those who reported migraine with visual symptoms had a 1.5-fold increase risk of ischemic stroke. Women without visual symptoms were not shown to be at increased risk.

The association between migraine and other stroke risk factors has also been examined in the literature. The risk of stroke in patients with migraine is shown to be increased approximately threefold by smoking. Oral contraceptive use is associated with a fourfold higher risk of stroke in migraine patients.

The possible relationship between migraine and stroke has driven investigations into neuroimaging studies involving patients with migraine. Many of these studies have shown an association of migraine with clinically silent white matter lesions. A meta-analysis by Swartz et al. (2004) demonstrated an odds ratio of 3.9 between migraine and white matter lesions. A case-control study by Kruit (2004) did not find an overall increased prevalence of cerebral infarcts in migraine patients compared with age- and sex-matched control subjects. However, there was an increased prevalence of deep-cerebellar white matter lesions.

Empiric and research data on migraine have also led to the observation that vascular dysfunction may extend to coronary arteries. This association has been debated for a number of years in the literature, with many studies failing to show an association. Recently, two prospective cohort studies found an association between migraine and ischemic heart disease. Data from the Women's Health Study (Kurth et al., 2006) indicated an association between migraine with aura and ischemic vascular events. Compared with women who did not report any history of migraine, women who reported migraine with aura had an approximately twofold increased risk of major cardiovascular disease, myocardial infarction, coronary revascularization, angina, and cardiovascular-associated death.

Migraine has recently been shown to be associated with an unfavorable cardiovascular disease profile. The General Epidemiology of Migraine Study, by Scher and colleagues (2005), found that when compared with control subjects, migraineurs are more likely to have hyperlipidemia and hypertension and to report an early onset of coronary artery disease. A recent study by Welch et al. (2006) showed elevation of C-reactive protein, a marker of cerebrovascular disease in migraine patients with and without aura.

Potential mechanisms relating migraines to vascular disease include arterial dissection, cardioembolism, and endothelial dysfunction. Arterial dissection is a well-recognized cause of stroke in the young and has been shown to have increased prevalence in those with migraine (Tzourio et al., 2002). This is thought to be due to elevations of serum elastase in migraineurs, as demonstrated by Tzourio and colleagues (2000).

There is increasing evidence that migraine may be a risk factor for endothelial dysfunction, thereby establishing a link with ischemic stroke and heart disease. Elevation of von Willebrand factor (VWF), a biomarker of endothelial dysfunction, has been shown to be significantly higher in migraineurs than in nonheadache control subjects during the interictal phase. Levels of VWF have also been shown to increase during a migraine attack, suggesting a relation of migraine to the development of endothelial dysfunction (Tietjen et al., 2001).

Another possible mechanism linking migraine to ischemic vascular disease may be cardioembolic events. Patent foramen ovale (PFO) has been found to be more common in young ischemic stroke patients with migraine. PFO has also been shown to be associated with migraine with aura in the absence of stroke. Hypotheses for the possible relationship between PFO and migraine include shunted microbubbles possibly triggering migraine by creating a surface for platelet activation, or release of vasoactive substances.

Some earlier studies have shown PFO closure to reduce migraine frequency, suggesting a possible causal relationship between the two (Post et al., 2004). The only prospective, randomized trial on the presence or absence of therapeutic effect of PFO closure to date is the Migraine Intervention with STARFlex Technology (MIST) trial (Tepper, Sheftell, and Bigal, 2007). The primary end point—complete resolution of headache—was not obtained in the study. A secondary end point indicates that 42% of patients had at least a 50% reduction of migraine days, compared with 23% of sham subjects ($p=0.038$). Serious adverse events did occur in 2 patients in the implantation group. Further prospective trials are needed to clarify whether there is a therapeutic effect of PFO closure on migraine and whether this potential benefit outweighs the risk of adverse events from the procedure.

References

Beckham JC, Krug LM, Penzien DB, et al. (1992). The relationship of ovarian steroids, headache activity and menstrual distress: A pilot study with female migraineurs. *Headache*, **32**: 292–297.

Bigal ME, Liberman JN, Lipton RB. (2006). Obesity and migraine: A population study. *Neurology*, **66**: 545–550.

Brandes JL. (2006). The role of estrogen in migraine. *Journal of the American Medical Association*, **295**: 1824–1830.

Breslau N, Lipton RB, Stewart WF, Schultz LR, Welch KM. (2003). Comorbidity of migraine and depression: Investigating potential etiology and prognosis. *Neurology*, **60**: 1308–1312.

Breslau N, Merikangas K, Bowden CL. (1994). Comorbidity of migraine and major affective disorders. *Neurology*, **44(10 Suppl 7):** S17–S22.

Breslau N, Schultz LR, Stewart WF, et al. (2000). Headache and major depression: Is the association specific to migraine? *Neurology*, **54**: 308–313.

Calhoun AH, Ford S. (2007). Behavioral sleep modification may revert transformed migraine to episodic migraine. *Headache*, **47**: 1178–1184.

Calhoun AH, Ford S, Finkel AG, Kahn KA, Mann JD. (2006). The prevalence and spectrum of sleep problems in women with transformed migraine. *Headache*, **46**: 604–610.

Cole J, Rothman KJ, Cabral HJ, Zhang Y, Farraye F. (2006). Migraine, fibromyalgia and depression among people with IBS: A prevalence study. *British Medical Council Gastroenterology*, **6**: 26–30.

Etminan M, Takkouche B, Isorna FC, Samii A. (2005). Risk of ischemic stroke in people with migraine: A systematic review and meta-analysis of observational studies. *British Journal of Medicine*, **330:** 63–65.

Facchinetti F, Neri I, Martignoni E, Fiorini L, Nappi G, Genazzani AR. (1993). The association of mentstrual migraine with the premenstrual syndrome. *Cephalalgia*, **13:** 422–425.

Facchinetti F, Tarabusi M, Nappi G. (1998). Premenstrual syndrome and anxiety disorders: A psychobiological link. *Psychotherapy and Psychosomatics*, **67:** 57–60.

Ferrero S, Pretta S, Bertoldi S, et al. (2004). Increased frequency of migraine among women with endometriosis. *Human Reproduction*, **19:** 2927–2932.

Hamelsky SW, Lipton RB. (2006). Psychiatric comorbidity of migraine. *Headache*, **46:** 1327–1333.

Holland PR, Akerman S, Goadsby PJ. (2005). Orexin 1 receptor activation attenuates neurogenic dural vasodilation in an animal model of trigeminovascular nociception. *The Journal of Pharmacology and Experimental Therapeutics*, **315:** 1380–1385.

Ifergane G, Buskila D, Simisevely N, Zeev K, Cohen H. (2005). Prevalence of fibromyalgia syndrome in migraine patients. *Cephalalgia*, **26:** 451–456.

Kelman L, Rains JC. (2005). Headache and sleep: Examination of sleep patterns and complaints in a large clinical sample of migraineurs. *Headache*, **45:** 904–910.

Kruit MC, van Buchem MA, Hofman PAM, et al. (2004). Migraine as a risk factor for subclinical brain lesions. *Journal of the American Medical Association*, **291(4):** 427–434.

Kurth T, Gaziano JM, Cook NR, et al. (2006). Migraine and risk of cardiovascular disease in women. *Journal of the American Medical Association*, **296:** 283–291.

Kurth T, Slomke MA, Kase CS, et al. (2005). Migraine, headache, and the risk of stroke in women: A prospective study. *Neurology*, **64:** 1573–1577.

Marcus DA, Bernstein C, Rudy TE. (2005). Fibromyalgia and headache: An epidemiological study supporting migraine as part of the fibromyalgia syndrome. *Clinical Rheumatology*, **24:** 595–601.

Martin V, Wernke S, Mandell K, et al. (2006). Symptoms of premenstrual syndrome and their association with migraine headache. *Headache*, **46:** 125–137.

McIntyre RS, Konarski JZ, Wilkins K, et al. (2006). The prevalence and impact of migraine headache in bipolar disorder: Results from the Canadian Community Health Survey. *Headache*, **46:** 973–982.

McWilliams L, Goodwin R, Cox B. (2004). Depression and anxiety associated with three pain conditions: Results from a nationally representative sample. *Pain*, **111(1–2):** 77–83.

Merikangas KR, Angst J, Isler H. (1990). Migraine and psychopathology. Results of the Zurich cohort study of young adults. *Archives of General Psychiatry*, **47(9):** 849–853.

Peterlin BL, Loder EW. (2006). Premenstrual headache: Diagnostic and pathophysiologic considerations. *Current Headache Reports*, **5:** 193–199.

Peterlin BL, Ward T, Lidicker J, Levin M. (2007a). A retrospective, comparative study on the frequency of abuse in migraine and chronic daily headache. *Headache*, **47:** 397–401.

Peterlin BL, Tietjen GE, Meng S, et al. (2007b). Post-traumatic stress disorder in episodic and chronic migraine. *Headache*, **6** (in press).

Peterlin BL, Bigl ME, Tepper SJ, Urakaze M, Sheftell FD, Rapoport AM. (2007c). Migraine and adiponectin: Is there a connection? *Cephalalgia*, **27:** 435–446

Post MC, Thijs V, Herroelen L, Budts WI. (2004). Closure of a patent foramen ovale is associated with a decrease in prevalence of migraine. *Neurology*, **62:** 1439–1440.

Rains JC, Poceta JS. (2006). Headache and sleep disorders: Review and clinical implications for headache management. *Headache*, **46:** 1344–1363.

Rasmussen BK. (1993). Migraine and tension type headache in a general population: Precipitating factors, female hormones, sleep pattern and relation to lifestyle. *Pain*, **53:** 65–72.

Sarchielli P, Filippo M. (2007). Sensitization, glutamate, and the link between migraine and fibromyalgia. *Current Pain and Headache Reports*, **11:** 343–351.

Scher AI, Terwindt GM, Picavet HSJ, Verschuren WMM, Ferrari MD, Launer LJ. (2005). Cardiovascular risk factors and migraine: The GEM population-based study. *Neurology*, **64:** 614–620.

Scher A, Lipton R, Stewart W. (2003a). Habitual snoring as a risk factor for chronic daily headache. *Neurology*, **60:** 1366–1368.

Scher AI, Stewart WF, Ricci JA, Lipton RB. (2003b). Factors associated with the onset and remission of chronic daily headache in a population-based study. *Pain*, **1061:** 81–89.

Seedat S, Stein DJ, Carey PD. (2005). Post-traumatic stress disorder in women: Epidemiological treatment issues. *CNS Drugs*, **19:** 411–427.

Swartz RH, Kern RZ. (2004). Migraine is associated with magnetic resonance imaging white matter abnormalities: A meta-analysis. *Archives of Neurology*, **61(9):** 1366–1368.

Tepper SJ, Sheftell FD, Bigal ME. (2007). The patent foramen ovale–migraine question. *Neurological Sciences*, **28 Suppl:** S118–S123.

Tietjen GE. (2007). Migraine and ischemic heart disease and stroke: Potential mechanisms and treatment implications. *Cephalagia*, **27:** 981–987.

Tietjen GE, Al Qasmi MM, Athanas K, Dafer RM, Khuder SA. (2001). Increased von Willebrand factor in migraine. *Neurology*, **57:** 334–336.

Tietjen GE, Brandes JL, Digre KB, Baggaley S, Martin V, Recober A. (2007a). High prevalence of somatic symptoms and depression in women with disabling chronic headache. *Neurology*, **68:** 134–140.

Tietjen GE, Bushnell C, Herial N, et al. (2007b). Endometriosis is associated with prevalence of comorbid conditions in migraine. *Headache*, **47:** 1069–1078.

Tietjen GE, Conway A, Utley C, Gunning WT, Herial NA. (2006). Migraine is associated with menorrhagia and endometriosis. *Headache*, **46:** 422–428.

Tietjen GE, Peterlin BL, Brandes JL, et al. (2007c). Depression and anxiety: Effect on the migraine-obesity relationship. *Headache*, **47(6):** 866–875.

Tzourio C, Benslamia L, Guillon B, et al. (2002). Migraine and the risk of cervical artery dissection: A case-control study. *Neurology*, **59:** 435–437.

Tzourio C, El Amrani M, Robert L, Alperovitch A. (2000). Serum elastase activity is elevated in migraine. *Annals of Neurology*, **47:** 648–651.

Welch KMA, Brandes AW, Salerno L, Brandes JL. (2006). C-reactive protein may be increase in migraine patients who present with complex clinical features. *Headache*, **46:** 197–199.

Chapter 6

Pharmacotherapy

E. Anne MacGregor

Acute treatment

The treatment of menstrually related attacks of migraine is, initially at least, the same as for nonmenstrual attacks. Optimal acute abortive treatment may be all that a woman requires. In practice, this means the use of an appropriate medication, taken in an adequate dose, at a mild stage of the attack, together with appropriate treatment of associated symptoms such as nausea or vomiting. Acute abortive treatment regimens usually include analgesics such as nonsteroidal anti-inflammatory drugs (NSAIDs), ergot derivatives, and triptans with or without prokinetic antiemetics (Steiner et al., 2007).

Over-the-counter drugs are appropriate agents only for the treatment of mild to moderate headache, provided patients get adequate benefit and do not overuse them. If patients do not obtain adequate relief from headache, prescription medications should be considered. Sedating or habit-forming medications such as those containing barbiturates, opioids, or caffeine should be avoided, as inappropriate use can result in dependency and medication-overuse headache. Multiple triptan studies, including one for almotriptan, eletriptan, frovatriptan, naratriptan, rizatriptan, sumatriptan, and zolmitriptan, have shown significant efficacy for acute abortive therapy of menstrually related migraine (MRM) attacks.

Continuous prophylaxis

Nonhormonal

Standard prophylactic pharmacotherapy

Standard prophylactic drugs, such as amitriptyline or topiramate, should be considered for women with MRM who also have frequent nonmenstrual attacks. If MRM remains refractory, specific strategies can be used subsequent to, or in conjunction with, standard prophylaxis.

Magnesium

Magnesium prolidone carboxylic acid 360 mg decreased the duration and intensity of premenstrual migraine in a small, placebo-controlled, double-blind study

Table 6.1 Acute pharmacotherapy
Analgesics ± prokinetic antiemetics
Nonsteroidal anti-inflammatory drugs
Ergot derivatives
Triptans

Table 6.2 Continuous prophylaxis
• Hormonal
• Continuous combined hormonal contraceptives
• Progestogen-only contraceptives
• Hormone replacement therapy
• Gonadotropin-releasing hormone analogues
• Dopamine agonists
• Antiestrogens
• Nonhormonal
• Standard prophylactic pharmacotherapy
• Magnesium

of women with premenstrual syndrome and migraine (Facchinetti et al., 1991). Diarrhea is the major side effect and can sometimes be controlled by changing preparation. Magnesium oxide is widely available, and the recommended dose is 300 to 600 mg daily.

Hormonal

Continuous combined hormonal contraceptives

Combined hormonal contraceptives inhibit ovulation by inhibiting both follicle-stimulating hormone (FSH) and luteinizing hormone (LH). Continuous hormones are recommended based on evidence that estrogen withdrawal during the hormone-free interval provokes headache and migraine in susceptible women (MacGregor and Hackshaw, 2002; Sulak et al., 2007). No double-blind, placebo-controlled trials of this strategy in menstrual migraine have been performed. However, one open-label study did show a reduction in daily headache scores after use of a 28-day extended placebo-free regimen, and this reduction persisted throughout the 168-day regimen (Sulak et al., 2007). Combined hormonal contraceptives should not be used by women with migraine with aura because of the synergistic increased risk of ischemic stroke (Faccinetti et al., 1991).

Progestogen-only contraceptives

Intramuscular depot medroxyprogesterone acetate (Depo Provera), subdermal etonogestrel (Implanon), and oral desogestrel (Cerazette) inhibit ovulation. Depot progestogens inhibit both FSH and LH; subdermal etonogestrel and oral desogestrel inhibit the LH surge, maintaining follicular phase estrogen activity. Irregular bleeding is often associated with migraine. The levonorgestrel intrauterine system (IUS) is highly effective at reducing menstrual bleeding and associated pain. It can be considered for migraine related to menorrhagia, particularly if the pain has responded to NSAIDs. Systemic effects are usually minor, but erratic bleeding and spotting are common in the early months of use. The IUS is not effective for women who are sensitive to estrogen withdrawal as a migraine trigger, as the majority of women still ovulate.

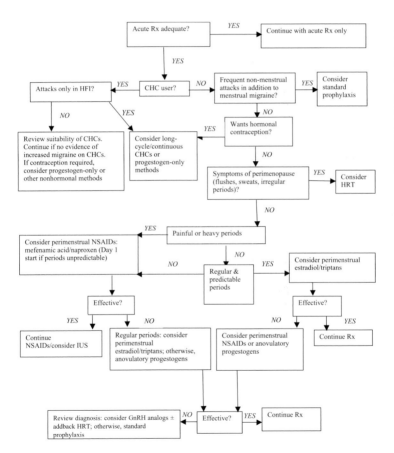

Figure 6.1 Algorithm for the management of menstrual attacks of migraine. CHC, combined hormonal contraceptives; GnRH, gonadotropin releasing hormone; HFI, hormone-free interval; HRT, hormone replacement therapy; IUS, intrauterine system; NSAIDs, nonsteroidal anti-inflammatory drugs. Adapted with permission, MacGregor EA, 2007.

Hormone replacement therapy

Perimenopause may mark a time of increased migraine. Hormone replacement therapy (HRT) can help, not only by stabilizing estrogen fluctuations associated with migraine but also by relieving night sweats, which often disturb sleep. HRT should only be started when periods become irregular and/or other menopausal symptoms such as hot flushes are present. Evidence from controlled trials supports earlier observations that HRT initiated during perimenopause is not associated with increased risk of stroke and cardiovascular disease and is more likely to have beneficial effects. Non-oral routes are preferred to oral formulations as they provide more stable estrogen levels (MacGregor, 2007).

Continuous combined HRT appears to be better tolerated by migraineurs than cyclical combined HRT. If oral preparations are favored, micronized estradiol is the preferred option as opposed to synthetic conjugated estrogen. If progesterone is needed in the case of an intact uterus, then micronized oral progesterone is recommended as opposed to synthetic progesterone. The minimum effective dose should be used, as too high a dose can trigger migraine aura (MacGregor, 1999).

Gonadotropin-releasing hormone analogues

By instigating a "medical" menopause, gonadotropin-releasing hormone (GnRH) analogues effectively abolish menstrual migraine (Holdaway et al., 1991). However, their use is limited by the effects of estrogen deficiency, such as hot flushes and reduction in bone density. "Add-back" continuous combined estrogen and progestogen can be given to counter these difficulties (Martin et al., 2003). Given these limitations and the high cost, such treatment should be instigated only in specialist departments.

Dopamine agonists

Bromocriptine inhibits GnRH and LH. Its use can result in reduced peak luteal phase estradiol levels and consequent reduced premenstrual estrogen withdrawal. Although small studies have suggested efficacy, there are no data from double-blind, placebo-controlled studies (Hockaday et al., 1976; Herzog, 1997).

Antiestrogens

Danazol has been used with some effect, but adverse effects restrict its use. Tamoxifen has been associated with a varying effect on migraine.

Practical recommendations for pharmacotherapy of menstrual migraine

Standard acute abortive agents to treat acute attacks may frequently be effective for women with MRM. If acute therapy alone is inadequate, preemptive treatment of the expected menstrual headache with short-term prophylaxis with NSAIDS, estradiol, or triptans is often an effective option.

For women whose headaches respond poorly to abortive treatment and for whom attempts at STP are not feasible or fail, or for those who have frequent nonmenstrual migraine, standard prophylactic agents taken throughout the cycle may be beneficial. More aggressive strategies should be restricted to therapeutic failures, and if these also fail, the diagnosis should be questioned.

Conclusions

- Effective acute abortive therapy is the mainstay of migraine management and may be all that is necessary to provide adequate control of MRM attacks.
- The choice of prophylaxis depends on the regularity of the menstrual cycle, timing of attack in relation to bleeding, presence of dysmenorrhea and/or menorrhagia, presence of perimenopausal symptoms, and need for contraception.

References

Facchinetti F, Sances G, Borella P, Genazzani AR, Nappi G. (1991). Magnesium prophylaxis of menstrual migraine: Effects on intracellular magnesium. *Headache*, **31:** 298–301.

Herzog AG. (1997). Continuous bromocriptine therapy in menstrual migraine. *Neurology*, **48:** 101–102.

Holdaway IM, Parr CE, France J. (1991). Treatment of a patient with severe menstrual migraine using the depot LHRH analogue Zoladex. *Australian New Zealand Journal of Obstetrics and Gynaecology*, **31:** 164–165.

Hockaday JM, Peet KM, Hockaday TD. (1976). Bromocriptine in migraine. *Headache*, **16:** 109–114.

MacGregor A. (1999). Estrogen replacement and migraine aura. *Headache*, **39:** 674–678.

MacGregor EA. (2007). Migraine, the menopause and hormone replacement therapy: A clinical review. *Journal of Family Planning and Reproductive Health Care*, **33:** 245–249.

MacGregor EA, Hackshaw A. (2002). Prevention of migraine in the pill-free interval of combined oral contraceptives: A double-blind, placebo-controlled pilot study using natural oestrogen supplements. *Journal of Family Planning and Reproductive Health Care*, **28:** 27–31.

Martin V, Wernke S, Mandell K, et al. (2003). Medical oophorectomy with and without estrogen add-back therapy in the prevention of migraine headache. *Headache*, **43:** 309–321.

Steiner TJ, MacGregor EA, Davies PTG. (2007). Guidelines for all healthcare professionals in the diagnosis and management of migraine, tension-type, cluster and medication overuse headache (3rd ed.). Available at: http://www.bash.org.uk. Accessed October 6, 2007.

Sulak P, Willis S, Kuehl T, Coffee A, Clark J. (2007). Headaches and oral contraceptives: Impact of eliminating the standard 7-day placebo interval. *Headache*, **47:** 27–37.

Chapter 7

Hormonal therapy and menstrual migraine: The estrogen controversy

Joan Golub and Susan Hutchinson

The use of estrogen in women with migraine has been controversial for years. Clinicians are often concerned that exogenous estrogen supplementation will aggravate migraines or increase the risk of ischemic stroke or venous thrombosis. However, we are dealing with a large population of women who are in their childbearing years; these women often need or want contraception. In other cases, hormone therapy may be warranted to control menstrual bleeding, menstrual irregularity, dysmenorrhea, endometriosis, or some of the disabling symptoms of perimenopause. This chapter will attempt to put into perspective the use of estrogen for women with migraine, and in particular menstrual migraine.

Estrogen pharmacology

The menstrual cycle is an intricately coordinated series of hormonal stimulations and suppressions designed to develop and release an ovum. Normal cycles can be 21 to 54 days apart, although the usual cycle is closer to 28 days (25 to 34 days apart). During the first part, the variable follicular phase, the ovary is the least hormonally active. The baseline estrogen and progesterone levels remain low. About 1 week before ovulation, follicular growth accelerates and the serum estrogen level rapidly rises, only to drop sharply as the dominant follicle releases and ovulation occurs. At ovulation, the 14-day luteal phase begins. The estrogen level starts to increase again; if no pregnancy occurs, then the estrogen level drops sharply several days before menstruation. It is these estrogen drops that can trigger migraine, with the latter a more significant trigger, as the "system" has been estrogen primed.

In the perimenopausal woman, the ovary is still active, but the normal pattern of estrogen and progesterone levels can vary greatly; in fact, many of the cycles can be "anovulatory." This irregularity can lead to highly variable bleeding patterns and unpredictability with menstrual migraine. Importantly, these women are still at risk of pregnancy. Estrogen-containing contraception is increasingly being used in this group, even as women approach 52 to 55 years of age (the average age of menopause is 51.5 years).

Estrogen and progestin are the components in "the Pill"; these we will refer to as combination oral contraceptives (COCs). In most of these COCs, the estrogen is ethinyl estradiol (E2), with the estrogen in a few of the older COCs being mestranol. Estradiol is the most potent natural estrogen, but it is not absorbed orally. Adding an ethinyl group at the 17 position makes it orally active. Mestranol is the 3-methyl ether of E2; it is weaker than E2 and must be converted to E2 before absorption. All of the low-dose COCs use E2. Low-dose COCs are products containing 35 µg or less of E2. The "mini pill" is a progestin-only contraceptive pill and is not discussed in this chapter. Combined hormonal contraceptives (CHCs) are available as dermal patches (Ortho Evra) and vaginal rings (Nuvaring) as well as COCs.

Low-dose COCs maintain the same high theoretical use as higher-dose COCs but may reduce troublesome side effects such as bloating, weight gain, nausea, and breast tenderness. Also, the lower-dose COCs may theoretically reduce one of the most serious side effects of COCs: thrombosis. Many clinicians believe the lower dose is the lowest dose that can be prescribed without sacrificing efficacy.

The COCs work in three ways:

1. Estrogen/progestin inhibition of the midcycle surge of gonadotropin secretion, thus preventing ovulation
2. Cause the cervical mucus to become hostile to sperm
3. Change the lining of the uterus to become hostile to implantation

It is the first mechanism that we are concerned with in this chapter.

Ovulation is stopped by inhibiting gonadotrophic secretion via an effect on both the hypothalamic and pituitary areas of the brain. Estrogen suppresses follicle-stimulating hormone (FSH), thereby stopping development of the dominant follicle. Progestin suppresses luteinizing hormone (LH) and ovulation.

Patient selection/risks

Hormonal contraception can be safely provided to most women after a careful medical history and blood pressure measurement. Breast exams, Pap smears, and sexually transmitted disease (STD) testing are encouraged but not required for initiation of a contraceptive pill, per the American College of Obstetricians and Gynecologists (ACOG) and the World Health Organization (WHO) (Stewart et al., 2001), but these procedures are usually performed in routine clinical practice. The same guidelines are used whether the COCs are used as contraception or for other medical indications.

Age alone is no longer a contraindication to COCs. The U.S. Food and Drug Administration (FDA) changed this in 1989, allowing COC through menopause for healthy nonsmokers. Cardiovascular disease is probably the most important issue to consider. Much of our current knowledge has been obtained through four major studies: the Royal College of General Practitioners (RCGP) Study, the Oxford Family Planning Association Study, the Walnut Creek Contraceptive Drug Study, and the Group Health Cooperative of Puget Sound Study. The RCGP study reported an increase in cardiovascular disease in women on COC over age 35 who smoked (Croft and Hannaford, 1989). Women smoking more than 15 cigarettes per day were at higher risk. Other studies have confirmed the increased risk of acute myocardial infarction in women who smoked or had hypertension and were on COCs (WHO, 1997). However, that risk increased significantly in older smoking women on COCs. A consensus panel reviewing the issue of oral contraception and smoking suggested that COCs can be used for fertile women over 35 years of age who are light smokers (fewer than 15 cigarettes per day) because the risks of pregnancy in this age group are greater than the risks associated with COC use (Schiff et al., 1999).

COCs often raise blood pressure; however, this is usually mild and within normal range. Overt hypertension can occur. The Nurses Health Study, a study of approximately 70,000 nurses aged 25 to 42 years, showed the relative risk of hypertension to be 1.8 for current COC uses compared with those who never used the Pill and 1.2 for previous users (Chasan-Taber et al., 1996). However, the risk quickly lowered when COCs were stopped. As hypertension and contraceptive users seem at high risk for acute myocardial infarction, recognition of hypertension is important.

The risk of stroke in COC users is an important cardiovascular risk. Most studies do not note an increase in hemorrhagic stroke; most studies do indicate a significant increase in ischemic stroke with COC users. This is particularly important as migraine is an independent risk factor for ischemic stroke; migraine with aura is an even greater risk for ischemic stroke. This has led both WHO and ACOG to list estrogen-containing contraception as contraindicated for women migraineurs who experience aura. Fortunately, the majority of women with migraine do not have aura; in fact, by definition, menstrual migraine is migraine without aura (Headache Classification Subcommittee of the International Headache Society, 2004).

Other important considerations and contraindications are acute liver disease, hormonally dependent cancer (e.g., breast), undiagnosed vaginal bleeding, and pregnancy.

Non-oral CHCs lessen the impact on acute liver disease, but the contraceptive patch is considered by many as high dose (equal to a 62 μg oral estrogen dose).

So who, then, is a candidate for estrogen-containing contraception? A practical approach would be to look at all the cardiac risk factors a woman has and then come to a treatment decision. Here are some practical considerations:

1. Does the woman smoke? If so, how many cigarettes a day?
2. What is her blood pressure?
3. Is she overweight?

4. What is her age if she has any of these higher-risk comorbidities?
5. Is there a personal or family history of heart disease, venous thrombosis, or clotting disorder? The risk of thrombosis is thought to be related to estrogen and not progestin. The higher the dose of estrogen, the greater the risk of thrombosis, theoretically. However, ACOG does not recommend prescreening patients for coagulopathies before initiation of estrogen-containing contraception. Factor V Leiden, the most common form of inherited thrombophilia, should be evaluated in prescreening if there is family history of phlebitis, pulmonary embolism, or stroke. Most authorities recommend avoiding estrogen-containing products in patients positive for this marker.
6. Does she have migraine? If so, does she ever experience aura? How often does she get aura? How long does it last? When did it last occur?

It is these authors' opinion that aura is overdiagnosed, especially when patients complain only of blurry vision or an occasional spot in their visual field. A vivid description of zig-zag lines across the visual field, scintillating lights, or loss of vision such as tunnel-vision are all suggestive of visual aura. Aura, by definition, refers to the reversible neurological signs and symptoms that typically occur 60 minutes or less before the headache.

Should a woman who occasionally experiences aura and has no other risk factors for stroke be allowed to take estrogen-containing contraception? There is no clear-cut answer here; ACOG and WHO guidelines say no. Many clinicians may allow such a woman to go on low-dose estrogen-containing contraception because the risks of pregnancy can be great. Educating the patient regarding her increased risk of ischemic stroke and documenting that discussion in the medical record would be recommended. Additionally, some neurologists would recommend a daily low-dose aspirin for these women. Last, these women should be followed closely and should report any new or prolonged aura symptoms that may necessitate stopping any estrogen.

Now, let's turn to look at specific hormonal therapies that are commonly used in women with menstrual migraine. Keep in mind that many of these women need or want contraception or hormone therapy; we are not suggesting that hormonal therapy is the mainstay of treatment for menstrual migraine. However, it makes sense to look at specific hormonal therapy in relationship to menstrual migraine. Are there some regimens that are theoretically better for the female migraineur?

Hormonal therapy and menstrual migraine

Hormonal therapy for migraine includes CHC, in which both estrogen and progesterone are in the formulation, and estrogen replacement therapy (ERT), in which estrogen alone may be used. Per Somerville's (1972) classic work, the use of progesterone therapy alone can delay menses and thus menstrual migraine, but it does not lessen the migraine. It is important to make a distinction between contraceptive doses of hormones versus replacement hormonal doses. Contraceptive doses suppress ovarian function, prevent ovulation and pregnancy, and are often referred to as providing "supra-physiological" doses of hormones. In contrast, hormonal therapy, such as with an estradiol 0.1 mg patch, does not suppress ovarian function, does not prevent pregnancy, and is a much more physiological dose of hormonal therapy. Importantly, a woman's own endogenous ovarian hormonal production is still occurring with the lower doses of noncontraceptive hormonal therapy. This distinction becomes important when deciding which hormonal therapy may be most appropriate for an individual patient.

Combined hormonal contraception

This hormonal treatment is most appropriate for those woman migraine patients who need contraception or need CHC to control bleeding, severe dysmenorrhea, and endometriosis, as well as perimenopausal symptoms. It is assumed for this section that women have been screened and are considered candidates for CHC—that is, they are nonsmokers, have no significant cardiac or stroke risk factors, and do not have migraine with aura. Which formulations would be most appropriate and least likely to aggravate their migraines? Can their migraines improve with certain contraceptive formulations? To answer these questions, let's first look at formulation options for estrogen-containing contraception (also known as CHC).

Formulation options for estrogen/progesterone contraception treatment include oral and nonoral routes of administration. Oral contraceptive formulations can be divided into monophasic or multiphasic (mainly triphasic); monophasic would indicate that the estrogen and progesterone content of all active pills is the same. In triphasic pills, the estrogen and/or progesterone content varies and is usually noted by a change in color in the pill pack. For years, oral contraceptive pills were packaged as 21 days (3 weeks) of the active pill followed by 1 week of the inactive or placebo pill. It was often during this week that women reported worsening of their migraines. Over recent years, there have been many new dosing regimens. These include the following:

1. **Continuous extended release contraception** (Seasonale)—12 weeks of active contraceptive pill followed by 1 week of placebo. A new preparation (Lybrel) of 90 μg levonorgestrel and 20 μg ethinyl estradiol is taken continuously with no placebo intervals.
2. **Add-back estrogen the week of the placebo**—3 weeks of 20 μg ethinyl estradiol; 2 days placebo; 5 days 10 μg ethinyl estradiol (Mircette). A new variation on this is continuous extended-release oral contraceptive pill of 30 μg ethinyl estradiol for 12 weeks followed by 1 week of ethinyl estradiol 10 μg (Seasonique).
3. **Extended dosing regimens**—24 active oral contraceptive pills followed by 4 days placebo (Yaz; Loestrin 24)

It can be very confusing to know exactly what the patient is taking from the name she may give you for her oral contraceptive; there are many generic formulations of commonly used regimens. Therefore, it is recommended that patients bring in their pill pack so that the provider can look at the specific amount of estrogen and progesterone in the pill pack and how the pill pack is packaged. Additionally, it can be very useful to have the woman point to where in her pill pack she has the most problems with her migraines. So, with all these formulations, what are some general guidelines that can be recommended for our female migraineurs?

Recommended guidelines for oral contraception
for female migraineurs

1. Use a monophasic pill containing 35 µg or less of ethinyl estradiol. Oral doses range from 20 to 35 µg of ethinyl estradiol for most commonly used formulations; all are considered "low dose." There are some data that 20 µg pills do not sufficiently suppress ovulation. Also, for women who weigh over 160 lb, the 35 µg ethinyl estradiol pills will give more protection than <35 µg.
2. Consider using the pill in a continuous fashion by minimizing any days of placebo.
3. Have the patient cycle off to have withdrawal bleeding only as needed. Most commonly, this is done every 3 months. This may need to be cleared with her treating gynecologist if that is not your role in her care.
4. Consider "add-back" estrogen when cycling off to minimize drops in estradiol, which can trigger menstrual migraine. This can be accomplished by using estradiol 0.1 mg patch; most women prefer name-brand patches to minimize skin irritation. Name-brand estradiol patches also tend to be smaller in size.

A key point is that the incidence of headache complaints has been reported to be 9.7% in women using extended-regimen OCs versus 17.3% in those using standard-regimen OCs (Cachrimandou et al., 1993). Although it was not determined whether these were migraine headaches, it would seem to indicate that extended regimens could be favorable for the migraine patient. Theoretically, the more steady-state level of estradiol made possible by eliminating the placebo week could lessen the severity and duration of menstrual migraine. It is commonly accepted that the drop in estradiol just prior to menses is a trigger for menstrual migraine; this drop can be exogenous from the transition from active to placebo on oral contraceptives. Preventing this drop in estradiol is a reasonable treatment strategy for the female migraine patient who suffers from menstrual migraine.

Nonoral estrogen-containing contraceptives

Nonoral estrogen-containing contraceptive options include the transdermal contraceptive patch (Ortho Evra) and the contraceptive vaginal ring (Nuvaring).

Caution is advised with the contraceptive patch because users may be exposed to 60% more estrogen than are women using a 35 µg ethinyl estradiol OC; in addition, the level of estradiol provided by the patch may not remain steady, and the peak value may be 25% lower than that experienced with OCs (Ortho Evra, 2007). The contraceptive vaginal ring delivers 15 µg ethinyl estradiol and can be left in continuously for 4 weeks. The ring would then be replaced every 4 weeks.

Noncontraceptive hormonal therapy

This type of treatment refers to the use of hormonal therapy in the form of estrogen for women migraineurs who do not need or want contraception, such as a woman who has had a tubal ligation or whose husband or partner has had a vasectomy. It has been found that a 0.1 mg transdermal estradiol patch applied perimenstrually can be effective in preventing menstrual migraine, whereas a 0.05 mg patch is ineffective (Pradalier et al., 1994). The data suggest that it may be necessary to maintain a serum estradiol level >45 pg/mL to prevent menstrual migraine, as the 0.1 mg patch produces serum estradiol levels of 45 to 75 pg/mL (Martin and Behbehani, 2006). Alternatively, oral estrogen can be given during the perimenstrual period, such as 0.9 mg/day of CEEs; this was shown to yield a 77% reduction in the number of headache days per cycle (Calhoun, 2004).

Many women are given transdermal estradiol patches during perimenopause by their gynecologist or primary care provider to help their vasomotor symptoms; they often wear the patch continuously. It is important to remember that these women are still experiencing variable levels of estrogen and progesterone from their own ovaries. The transdermal estradiol patch is simply providing a "layer" of estradiol to help with symptoms. This regimen is not geared toward helping menstrual migraine.

Monitoring hormonal therapy in women with menstrual migraine

Once hormonal therapy in the form of combined contraception or supplemental estradiol is begun in a woman with migraine, how often should the woman be seen? This may vary depending on the age of the patient, the presence of any risk factors, and the provider's clinical opinion. In general, the younger and healthier the patient, the less often she needs to return. However, all women with migraine should be *strongly encouraged* to keep a headache diary as hormone therapy is initiated to see if her migraines worsen, improve, or remain unchanged. The woman migraine patient should include the first and last days of menses on her headache diary. The following are some general guidelines for follow-up of the female migraine patient on hormones:

1. Monitor blood pressure.
2. Monitor weight.
3. Ask about any new cardiac risk factors that may develop between visits.
4. Review the headache calendar: look for any worsening of headache, any new aura, and any worsening of prior aura symptoms. New aura or worsening of

aura would be indications to stop estrogen therapy. Worsening of headaches would indicate a need to reevaluate the current hormonal management.

As a headache clinician, I like to see women migraine patients back within 2 months of any change in hormonal therapy. Once it is established that a particular hormonal regimen is not aggravating her prior pattern of migraine, less frequent office visits may be appropriate. Also, the need or reasons to stay on a particular hormonal regimen can be discussed at all follow-up visits.

Conclusion

An estimated 12 million women suffer from menstrual migraines annually (Granella et al., 1993). These women are of childbearing age and often desire contraception; others may need estrogen-containing contraception or hormonal therapy for conditions such as endometriosis, dysmenorrhea, menorrhagia, or acne and for the relief of perimenopausal symptoms. We hope this chapter has helped put into perspective the use of estrogen for women with migraine.

References

Cachrimandou AC, Hellberg D, Nilsson S, et al. (1993). Long-interval treatment regimen with desogestrel-containing oral contraceptive. *Contraception*, **48 (3):** 205–216.

Calhoun AH. (2004). A novel specific prophylaxis for menstrual-associated migraine. *Southern Medical Journal*, **97(9):** 819–822.

Chasan-Taber L, Willett WC, Manson JE, et al. (1996). Prospective study of oral contraceptives and hypertension among women in the United States. *Circulation*, **94:** 483.

Croft P, Hannaford PC. (1989). Risk factors for acute myocardial infarction in women: Evidence from the Royal College of General Practioners' Oral Contraception Study. *BMJ*, **298:** 165.

Granella F, Sances G, Zanferrari C, et al. (1993). Migraine without aura and reproductive life events: A clinical epidemiological study in 1300 women. *Headache*, **33:** 385–389.

Important safety information. (n.d.). Ortho Evra Web site. Available at: http://www.orthoevra.com/html/pevr/safety.jsp;jsessionid=U5D02BQ0I1L54CQPCCEDCOYKB2IIWNSC? Accessed January 17, 2007.

Headache Classification Subcommittee of the International Headache Society. (2004). The international classification of headache disorders: 2nd edition. *Cephalalgia*, **24(Suppl 1):** 9–160.

Martin VT, Behbehani M. (2006). Ovarian hormones and migraine headaches: Understanding mechanisms and pathogenesis: Part 2. *Headache*, **46(3):** 365–386.

Pradalier A, Vincent D, Beaulieu P, et al. (1994). Correlation between oestradiol plasma level and therapeutic effect on menstrual migraine. In Rose FC (ed.), *New Advances in Headache Research* (4th ed., pp. 129–132). London: Smith-Gordon.

Schiff I, Bell WR, Davis V, et al. (1999). Oral contraceptives and smoking, current considerations: Recommendations of a consensus panel. *American Journal of Obstetrics and Gynecology*, **180:** S383.5.

Somerville BW. (1972). The role of estradiol withdrawal in the etiology of menstrual migraine. *Neurology*, **22(4):** 355–365.

Stewart FH, Harper CC, Ellertson CE, et al. (2001). Clinical breast and pelvic examination requirements for hormonal contraception: Current practice vs evidence. *Journal of the American Medical Association*, **285:** 2232.

WHO Collaborative Study of Cardiovascular Disease and Steroid Hormone Contraception. (1997). Acute myocardial infarction and combined oral contraceptives: Results of an international multicentre case-control study. *The Lancet*, **349:** 1202.

Chapter 8

Nonpharmacological interventions for the management of menstrually related migraine

Dawn C. Buse

The U.S. Headache Consortium developed evidence-based guidelines for the treatment and management of migriane headache based on extensive review of the medical literature and compilation of expert consensus. Published guidelines include data and recommendations on utility of nonpharmacological (behavioral and physical) treatments among other issues on the topics of migraine diagnosis and management (Campbell et al., 2000). A number of nonpharmacological treatments have empirical validation in treating migraine and other types of headaches and may also augment the effectiveness of other treatments or minimize the need for their use. Some patients may find that pharmacological treatments do not sufficiently manage their headache, and they may benefit from the addition of biobehavioral approaches. Others may want or need to avoid medication, such as women who are pregnant or trying to conceive (Scharff et al., 1996).

Nonpharmacological approaches offer the benefit of being cost effective without entailing potential drug interactions or side effects. However, physicians and patients should carefully review the evidence on the efficacy of nonpharmacological treatments, as well as the potential financial costs, lost treatment opportunities, and any potential adverse effects, before prescribing, recommending, or initiating their use. Nonpharmacological treatments for migraine can be divided into the categories of cognitive-behavioral therapy (CBT), biobehavioral training (i.e., biofeedback, relaxation training, and stress management), physical therapies, education, and lifestyle modification or "healthy lifestyle" training (Goslin et al., 1999; Campbell et al., 2000; Schwartz and Andrasik, 2003). Some techniques can be used by physicians during an appointment (e.g., diaphragmatic breathing and guided imagery), some can be self-taught and practiced by the patient (e.g., relaxation practice and stress management), and others such as biofeedback and CBT require a referral to an appropriately trained professional (e.g., psychologist; occupational therapist; social worker; or other licensed, experienced allied health professional.) There are also tools that can be helpful, such as educational books, Web sites, and other media, as well as support groups. Nonpharmacological approaches such as biobehavioral treatments may be offered individually or in conjunction with pharmacotherapy as part of a comprehensive treatment plan.

Biobehavioral treatments

"Biobehavioral treatment" refers to biofeedback, relaxation training, CBT, and stress management. Research has shown that these techniques can be very effective when practiced correctly and can be valuable additions to a pharmacological treatment plan (Campbell et al., 2000). Several behavioral treatments have demonstrated empirical efficacy for headache management and have become standard components of specialty headache centers and multidisciplinary pain management programs. Certain empirically validated biobehavioral approaches to headache management are endorsed by the American Medical Association, the World Health Organization, and the National Institutes of Health, as well as many other professional organizations (Goslin et al., 1999).

Biofeedback

Biofeedback is a behavioral intervention that involves monitoring physiological processes of which the patient is not consciously aware or does not believe that he or she has control. Biofeedback training is the process of increasing awareness of involuntary physiological functions and bringing them under voluntary control (Penzien and Holroyd, 1994; Schwartz and Andrasik, 2003). Biofeedback can be as effective as medication treatment for the prevention of many forms of primary headache. Typically, a patient is connected to biofeedback equipment to measure key physiological processes such as muscle tension, finger temperature, or heart rate. Physiological information is converted into a signal that is then "fed back" to the patient. Patients can monitor these processes through something as simple as a thermometer or as sophisticated as a computer screen with complex graphics. Patients then practice specific strategies such as diagrammatic breathing or visualization to induce the relaxation response or activation, which includes relaxation of the sympathetic nervous system and activation of the parasympathetic nervous system.

There are several biofeedback modalities, including thermal (finger temperature), muscular (electromyography [EMG]), and neurological or brain wave (electroencephalography [EEG]). Thermal biofeedback has been demonstrated to be most effective for the management of migraine, and EMG biofeedback is most effective for the management of tension-type headache. There is little empirical evidence regarding EEG biofeedback training. The *Evidence-Based Guidelines for Migraine Headache: Behavioral and Physical Treatments* (Campbell et al., 2000) gave Grade A status (meaning that the "quality of evidence was based on multiple well-designed randomized clinical trials, directly relevant to the recommendation, yielded a consistent pattern of findings") to relaxation training, thermal biofeedback combined with relaxation training, EMG biofeedback, and CBT as treatment options for prevention of migraine. They also reported that relaxation training and thermal biofeedback can produce 33% to 37% improvement in headache activity.

Thermal biofeedback, also known as "hand warming" biofeedback, involves monitoring finger temperature with a sensitive thermometer. The goal is for the patient to learn to raise finger temperature. Finger temperature is a measure of circulation. As sympathetic activity increases, circulation to the extremities decreases and finger temperature decreases. As parasympathetic activity increases and the relaxation response is activated, circulation and extremity temperature increase; therefore, higher finger temperature corresponds to a more relaxed state. EMG biofeedback involves monitoring muscle tension, usually in the head or neck area, with the goal of learning to lower muscle tension. EMG biofeedback is especially effective for reducing the microvoltage in tense muscles that is commonly associated with migraine, chronic tension-type headache, and cervicogenic headache.

Biofeedback generally requires several office visits (between 6 and 12) spaced 1 to several weeks apart. Providers are often psychologists who incorporate cognitive-behavioral techniques into sessions. Patients are taught techniques in the office; however, home practice is also required between sessions. As the patient's ability to manipulate and control the targeted physiological processes increases, the biofeedback device can be eliminated. One of the biggest challenges for physicians and patients can often be locating a biofeedback practitioner. The Association for Applied Psychophysiology and Biofeedback (AAPB) (www.aapb.org) is a professional organization for those certified to conduct biofeedback training, although many psychologists practice biofeedback therapy without being certified or belonging to this organization. A list of practitioners can be found at the Web site of the Biofeedback Certification Institute of America (BCIA) (www.bcia.org/directory/membership.cfm). A list of psychologists, along with their specialties and location, can be found at www.apa.org (telephone: 800-964-2000) or www.nationalregister.org. For additional information and to find practitioners in Europe, you may refer to the Biofeedback Foundation of Europe (www.bfe.org). A self-training biofeedback kit with an instructional CD-ROM and finger thermometer is available from www.headachecare.com (telephone 800-769-7565) or www.cliving.org.

Relaxation techniques

Relaxation techniques can be used to minimize physiological responses to stress and decrease sympathetic arousal. These techniques are usually taught by psychologists or other mental health or allied pain professionals but can also be self-taught by patients through reading, listening to relaxation CDs, or audiotapes. Although they can be learned during sessions in the office, they require regular practice in order to become effective, automatic responses. Relaxation training may include breathing techniques such as diaphragmatic breathing, visual imagery, meditation, prayer, yoga, listening to music, self-hypnosis, listening to guided-relaxation CDs or tapes, and other methods of calming the mind and body (Hammond, 1990; Penzien and Holroyd, 1994).

Cognitive-behavioral therapy

CBT is an empirically validated treatment approach that helps patients identify behaviors that may increase or maintain headaches (including triggers and lifestyle habits) and maladaptive or dysfunctional targeting thoughts and responses to stress (Beck et al., 1979). Targets of CBT may include enhancing self-efficacy, assertiveness training, increasing coping skills, cognitive restructuring, and awareness of catastrophizing. These interventions aid in headache management by making patients more aware of triggers, including the relationship between stress and headache, and by identifying and challenging counterproductive or self-defeating beliefs and ideas. For example, a patient may be asked to identify psychological or behavioral factors that trigger or aggravate their headaches or may be challenged about beliefs that lead to feelings of hopelessness, helplessness, depression, and anxiety. This awareness allows the patient to make use of more effective coping mechanisms and to increase self-efficacy. CBT is also used to manage and reduce feelings of depression, anxiety, panic attacks, obsessive-compulsive disorder, eating disorders, sleep disorders, and common comorbidities for headache sufferers.

Patients should work with a licensed psychologist, psychiatrist, or social worker with experience treating patients with headache or chronic medical conditions. For more information about CBT, go to the Association for Behavioral and Cognitive Therapies Web site at www.aabt.org. A list of psychologists by location and specialty may be found at www.apa.org (telephone: 800-964-2000) or www.nationalregister.org.

Education and lifestyle modification

In general, the best advice is for migraineurs to maintain a regular and healthy lifestyle, especially during times when they are most vulnerable to an attack. That includes a regular sleep/wake schedule; a regular and healthy diet; regular exercise; avoidance of excessive caffeine or alcohol consumption; smoking cessation; and regular practice of stress management, relaxation techniques, and self-care.

Patients with menstrually related migraine (MRM) have the advantage of knowing one of their most potent triggers and being able to predict or even preempt MRM attacks on a fairly regular monthly basis. Migraine is a predictable process. The prodrome provides a window of opportunity in which to use behavioral tools as a way to stop the process of migraine early, even before headache. Biobehavioral tools may also be used prophylactically and practiced on a regular basis in order to maintain homeostasis and manage stress so that the patient does not trigger a headache attack in the first place. Patients should be educated that during the week preceding and at the beginning of menses, they are most vulnerable to an attack. During this time period, they need to be especially aware of potential triggers, avoid stress, engage in relaxing and nurturing activities, and maintain a very regular and healthy lifestyle.

It is important for patients to use a diary to note associations. Some triggers cannot be changed or avoided, such as the menstrual cycle, in which case patients should be aware of their vulnerability to headache during this time and protect themselves by following a very healthy lifestyle. By doing so, they may reduce the number of headache attacks, although it is unlikely that the attacks will disappear altogether. Other triggers may be able to be eliminated or modified by patients. Discussed next are some of the most common headache triggers other than hormonal factors.

Diet and nutrition

Delayed, missed, or inadequate meals; caffeine consumption or withdrawal; dehydration; and certain foods (e.g., aged cheeses, chocolate, red wine, caffeinated drinks) may be triggers. Some patients may become overly focused on particular foods or may restrict their diet when it is not necessary. The most important information for migraineurs is to eat appropriately, regularly, and healthily; to try to avoid overly processed foods, foods with chemical additives and preservatives, and caffeine; and to maintain a healthy weight.

Sleep

Changes in sleep patterns and too little or too much sleep can be problematic. Migraineurs should maintain a regular sleep/wake schedule, even on weekends, going to bed and rising at the same time each day and ensuring enough hours of sleep per night. Patients should be educated on healthy sleep hygiene strategies.

Environmental factors

Many environmental factors can be problematic, including bright or flickering lights, strong smells, marked weather changes, changes in time zone, and work environment. Patients may or may not have control over these factors. If they are able to make modifications to these factors, that is best; otherwise, they should be aware of these potential triggers and try to avoid them if possible during times of vulnerability to attack.

Psychological and emotional factors

Stress, depression, anxiety, and other psychological and emotional factors are all related to migraine. While it may not be possible to control circumstances, we do have control over how we respond to them. Patients can be taught ways to modify thoughts, feelings, and behavior with CBT. They can be taught to manage the physiological effects of stress with biofeedback and relaxation training. Family members may also benefit from being educated about the effect of stress on migraine and may be made aware of the patient's need to avoid stress and take good care of herself during times of vulnerability to attack (e.g., a patient may tell her family that she must practice yoga and get enough sleep during the week preceding her period.) Paradoxically, some people will experience "letdown" headaches, which occur during the period of relaxation following a stressful period.

Protective factors

A migraineur has a sensitive nervous system that benefits from a stable and healthy routine including the activities mentioned earlier. In addition, research has demonstrated that migraine is related to a drop in serotonin levels in the brain (Goadsby et al., 2002). Certain activities are serotonin enhancing, including physical exercise; watching a funny movie or reading a funny book; spending time with a friend; receiving a massage, affection, or sexual activity; engaging in a hobby or pleasant activity; and biofeedback/relaxation (Cady and Shealy, 1989). By engaging in pleasant and self-nurturing activities, an individual creates a protective environment that balances the nervous system and lessens the potential vulnerability to an attack.

Support groups

Social support, whether through informal conversation in the physician's waiting room or organized support groups, can be extremely valuable. Patients often appreciate talking with someone else who "truly understands" and having the opportunity to speak with others outside of their family and regular social circle about how headaches affect their lives. Many countries and states have national headache associations that sponsor support groups. These organizations provide useful advice on how to cope with headache and put patients in contact with other headache sufferers in their area. The National Headache Foundation (NHF) has support groups listed by state on their Web site (www.headaches.org—or contact the Headache Education and Support Group and Membership Services Coordinator at 1-888-643-5552). They also offer an e-mail pen-pal program and message board. The American Headache Society (AHS) also offers support groups throughout the United States. For more information, visit their Web site at achehq@talley.com or call 1-800-255-2243. NHF and AHS will also assist patients in starting new support groups in their geographic area. Patients may find many other sites on the Internet; however, these sites may be supported by groups trying to profit from people with headache and/or may contain information that is not valid or reliable. Advise patients to contact one of the medical societies or other reputable organizations.

Physical treatments: Acupuncture, physical and occupational therapy, and massage

Data on the efficacy of physical treatments for migraine are limited by small sample size, poor study design, and weak results (Biondi, 2005). Physicians and patients are advised to make cautious and individualized judgments about the utility of physical treatments for migraine treatment and management. In some cases, these modalities may provide valuable additions to first-line pharmacological and biobehavioral treatment; however, cost, time, and potential adverse effects should be weighed carefully.

Acupuncture

Acupuncture is a component of the Chinese system of health care and can be traced back at least 2500 years. Acupuncture is based on the theory that there are patterns of energy (*Qi*) that flow through the body. The flow of *Qi* is essential for health, and disruptions of this flow are believed to be responsible for disease and pain. Data on the efficacy of acupuncture for migraine treatment and management are mixed. The National Institutes of Health (NIH) Consensus Development Program issued the following statement in 1997: "Acupuncture as a therapeutic intervention is widely practiced in the United States. There have been many studies of its potential usefulness. However, many of these studies provide equivocal results because of design, sample size, and other factors. The issue is further complicated by inherent difficulties in the use of appropriate controls, such as placebo and sham acupuncture groups" (NIH, 1998 [statement is available at http://consensus.nih .gov]). More recent meta-analyses and systematic reviews echo the same sentiments: while some research shows positive efficacy, the quality of research and, therefore, the ability to draw conclusions remain unclear at this time.

Physical and occupational therapy

A supervised physical therapy program of reconditioning and therapeutic exercise can provide benefits on many levels for patients who may not have the knowledge or motivation or who may not be physically capable of engaging in regular physical exercise on their own. Exercise improves physical functioning; may reduce body mass index; may reduce the somatic and cognitive experience of pain; has a beneficial impact on depression, anxiety, and feelings of self-worth; and aids in restoration of regular sleep/wake and eating cycles. A structured review of data on physical treatments for headache through 2004 reported that physical therapy is more effective than massage therapy or acupuncture for the treatment of headache and is most effective when combined with other treatments such as biofeedback, relaxation training, and exercise (Biondi, 2005).

The impact of chronic pain, including migraine headache, on daily life can be severe, even during the interictal periods (i.e., time between attacks) (Buse et al., 2007). Occupational therapists can help patients incorporate effective pain management strategies into activities of everyday life. Specific strategies can include goal setting, group programs, pacing techniques, assertive communication, use of appropriate body mechanics during everyday activities, and assistive devices or environmental modifications to support independent function. Both physical and occupational therapy are aimed at increasing patients' use of independent pain management modalities and reducing disability and dependence on medication.

Patients with chronic diseases with episodic manifestations such as migraine may remain in bed or do very little on days when pain is particularly severe and then compensate with intense overactivity on days when they are pain free. This leads to a sense of frustration on the part of the patient and makes it difficult to participate reliably in work, social, and vocational or educational activities. Occupational therapists work with patients to identify such patterns and concentrate on pacing techniques. These emphasize avoidance of large swings in activity levels and encourage the use of frequent breaks in activity regardless of pain level, as well as the incorporation of active pain control techniques on a regular basis to prevent pain escalation. These techniques include the development of a schedule that incorporates such things as the use of heat, ice, and relaxation strategies into the daily routine. Scheduled use of pain control modalities can enhance the effectiveness of other therapeutic and pharmacological interventions. Use of these strategies and progress toward desired activities and goals can be monitored through the use of graphs or charts. As progress occurs, particularly if it is without large increases in pain, patients are able to directly observe the benefits. Patients can also be "rewarded" for pain self-management practices by incorporating pleasurable activities into these routines.

Massage

Few data exist on the efficacy of massage as a treatment for migraine. However, two studies found that massage led to reduction in migraine frequency and improvement in sleep quality when compared with control participants (Lawler and Cameron, 2006). The authors also observed beneficial effects on perceived stress and coping efficacy and noted that during sessions, massage induced decreases in state anxiety, heart rate, and cortisol.

Conclusion

Nonpharmacological approaches to headache treatment and management are valuable tools in the comprehensive management of patients suffering from MRM. Empirically validated treatments include CBT, biobehavioral training (i.e., biofeedback, relaxation training, and stress management), education, and lifestyle modification or "healthy lifestyle" training. Behavioral management of headache should be recommended as a standard treatment either in addition to or instead of pharmacological treatment for all patients who suffer from headache throughout all stages of life. Migraine commonly first occurs in adolescence or early adulthood. By encouraging patients to train their physiology through biofeedback and relaxation, adopt healthy lifestyle habits, and recognize and mediate the effects of stress in their lives, the physician is giving patients a set of tools that will last a lifetime.

References

Beck AT, Rush AJ, Shaw BF, Emery G. (1979). *Cognitive Therapy of Depression.* New York: Guilford Press, pp. 142–166.

Biondi DM. (2005). Physical treatments for headache: A structured review. *Headache: The Journal of Head and Face Pain,* **45:** 738–746.

Buse DC, Bigal ME, Rupnow MFT, et al. (2007). The Migraine Interictal Burden Scale (MIBS): Results of a population-based validation study. *Headache*, **47:** 778.

Cady RK, Shealy CN. (1989). *Serotonin-Enhancing Activities and Pain Management.* Platform presentation, Southern Medical Association Annual Meeting, San Antonio, TX.

Campbell JK, Penzien DB, Wall EM. (2000). *Evidence-Based Guidelines for Migraine Headache: Behavioral and Physical Treatments.* US Headache Consortium. Available at: http://www.aan.com. Accessed October 19, 2007.

Goadsby PJ, Lipton RB, Ferrari MD. (2002). Migraine—current understanding and treatment. *New England Journal of Medicine*, **346:** 257–270.

Goslin RE, Gray RN, McCrory DC, et al. (1999). *Behavioral and physical treatments for migraine headache.* Technical review 2.2, February 1999. Prepared for the Agency for Health Care Policy and Research under Contract No. 290–94–2025. Available at: http://www.clinpol.mc.due.edu. Accessed January 14, 2006.

Hammond DC. (1990). *Handbook of Hypnotic Suggestions and Metaphors.* London: W. W. Norton.

Lawler SP, Cameron LD. (2006). A randomized, controlled trial of massage therapy as a treatment for migraine. *Annals of Behavioral Medicine*, **32:** 50–59.

NIH Consensus Conference. (1998). Acupuncture. *The Journal of the American Medical Association*, **280:** 1518–1524.

Penzien DB, Holroyd KA. (1994). Psychosocial interventions in the management of recurrent headache disorders—II: Description of treatment techniques. *Behavioral Medicine*, **20:** 64–73.

Scharff L, Marcus DA, Turk DC. (1996). Maintenance of effects in the nonmedical treatment of headaches during pregnancy. *Headache*, **36:** 285–290.

Schwartz MS, Andraski F. (eds.). (2003). *Biofeedback: A Practitioner's Guide* (3rd ed.). New York: Guilford Press.

Chapter 9

Conclusion

Susan Hutchinson and B. Lee Peterlin

The injuries that befall us unexpectedly are less severe than those which are deliberately anticipated.
—Marcus Tulius Cicero (great Roman writer and orator, 106–43 BC)

Although Cicero was not referring to menstrually related migraine, it is readily applicable. Migraine in itself is a common, chronic neurovascular disorder presenting as recurrent attacks of headache, which are often associated with substantial disability. It occurs in three times as many women as men. In addition, more than 50% of women notice that migraines are more likely to occur around menstruation. Menstrually related migraine attacks have been reported to be more severe and of longer duration than those outside of the perimenstrual period. And although the full pathophysiology of menstrually related migraine is not known, the excitability of cell membranes, which at least in part may be genetically determined, determines the brain's susceptibility to attacks. Factors that increase or decrease neuronal excitability modulate the threshold for triggering attacks. Estrogen withdrawal is one such migraine trigger—one that is potentially modifiable.

Knowledge of the International Classification of Headache Disorders and simple direct questions in regard to the temporal association of headache with menses in conjunction with headache calendars will help direct you to a correct diagnosis of menstrually related migraine. With a correct diagnosis, there are several therapeutic options in addition to traditional choices that can be successfully used in a woman with menstrually related migraine. In addition to non-pharmacological options and acute migraine therapy, in women with predictable menstrual cycles, short-term prophylaxis may be used. Short-term prophylaxis can be successfully accomplished with several options, including hormones, magnesium, naproxen sodium, and triptans. In those women with unpredictable menstrual cycles or refractory headaches, traditional preventive options should be used.

By providing education, support, and the most appropriate care available to a woman, physicians can build trust and truly establish therapeutic alliances with their patients. It is in this manner that we can help stop recurring, predictable, menstrually related migraine attacks and help provide women with the opportunity to gain control of their lives and step out of the shadow of pain.

Appendix A

ICHD-II Migraine Criteria

1.1 Migraine without aura

At least 5 attacks fulfilling the following 4 criteria:

1. Headache attacks lasting 4 to 72 hours (untreated or unsuccessfully treated)
2. Headache has at least 2 of the following characteristics:
   a. Unilateral location
   b. Pulsating quality
   c. Moderate or severe pain intensity
   d. Worsens with or causes avoidance of routine physical activity (e.g., Walking, climbing stairs)
3. During headache, at least one of the following symptoms is present:
   a. Nausea or vomiting
   b. Photophobia and phonophobia
4. Headache cannot be attributed to another disorder.

1.2.1 Typical aura with migraine headache

At least 2 attacks fulfilling the following 4 criteria:

1. Aura consisting of at least one of the following, but no motor weakness:
   a. Fully reversible visual symptoms including positive features (e.g., flickering lights, spots, or lines) and/or negative features (e.g., loss of vision)
   b. Fully reversible sensory symptoms including positive features (e.g., pins and needles) and/or negative features (e.g., numbness)
   c. Fully reversible dysphasic speech disturbance
2. At least 2 of the following:
   a. Homonymous visual symptoms and/or unilateral sensory symptoms
   b. At least one aura symptom developing gradually over at least 5 minutes and/or different aura symptoms occurring in succession for >5 minutes
   c. Each symptom lasts at least 5 minutes and no more than 60 minutes
3. Headache fulfilling all 4 criteria for 1.1 Migraine without aura begins during the aura or follows the aura within 60 minutes.
4. Headache cannot be attributed to another disorder.

Pure menstrual migraine

1.1 Migraine without aura occurring in at least 66% of menstrual cycles and exclusively during the 5-day perimenstrual period from day − 2 through +3 (day 1 = the first day of flow)

Menstrually related migraine

1.1 Migraine without aura occurring in at least 66% of menstrual cycles during the 5-day perimenstrual period from day − 2 through + 3 but also at other times during the cycle

2.1 Infrequent episodic tension-type headache

At least 10 episodes occurring on <1 day/month on average (<12 days/year) and fulfilling the following 3 criteria:

1. Headache lasting from 30 minutes to 1 hour
2. Headache has at least 2 of the following:
   a. Bilateral location
   b. Pressing/tightening (nonpulsating) quality
   c. Mild or moderate intensity
   d. Not aggravated by routine physical activity (such as walking or climbing stairs)
3. Both of the following:
   a. No nausea or vomiting (anorexia may be present)
   b. No more than 1 of photophobia or phonophobia

2.3 Chronic tension-type headache

Headache occurring on 15 or more days/month on average for >3 months and fulfilling all the above criteria except that headache may last for hours or may be continuous.

8.2 Medication overuse headache (MOH)

Headache present for >15 days/month and fulfilling the following criteria:

1. Intake of:
   a. Opioids and simple analgesics >15 days/month for >3 months
   b. Ergots, triptans, and combination analgesics >10 days/month for >3 months

2. Headache has developed or markedly worsened during the use of abortive medications.
3. Headache resolves or reverts to its previous pattern within 2 months after discontinuation of abortive medication.

Adapted from Headache Classification Subcommittee of the International Headache Society. (2004). The international classification of headache disorders: 2nd edition. *Cephalalgia*, **24(Suppl 1):** 9–160.

Appendix B

NECH HEADACHE CALENDAR*

Your Name: _____ Month: _____ Year: _____

HEADACHE SEVERITY   The calendar is numbered 1 – 31 for each day of the month. On the days you have headache pain, record in the box the number that describes your headache pain: 1 = mild; 2 = moderate; 3 = severe.

Day of Month	1	2	3	4	5	6	7	8	9	10	11	12	13	14	15	16	17	18	19	20	21	22	23	24	25	26	27	28	29	30	31
Morning																															
Afternoon																															
Evening/Night																															

Day of Month	1	2	3	4	5	6	7	8	9	10	11	12	13	14	15	16	17	18	19	20	21	22	23	24	25	26	27	28	29	30	31
MENSTRUAL PERIODS§																															
DISABILITY FOR THE DAY†																															

† **Disability**
Write a number from 0 to 3 that describes how your headache pain affected your activities for the day:
0 = no effect; 1 = able to carry out your activities fairly well; 2 = you had difficulty with usual activities and cancelled less important ones; 3 = you missed work for at least half the day or stayed in bed for part of the day.

§ **Menstrual Periods**
Place an "X" on the days you have your period.

ACUTE MEDICINES
(Medicines to treat headaches and related symptoms)

On the days you take medicines to relieve your headache pain write the names of the medicines and the doses in the appropriate box. Place a check (✓) for each dose you take. Also, record a number from 0 to 3 that describes the amount of overall relief you got from the medicine: 0 = no relief; 1 = slight relief; 2 = moderate relief; 3 = complete relief.

Day of Month	1	2	3	4	5	6	7	8	9	10	11	12	13	14	15	16	17	18	19	20	21	22	23	24	25	26	27	28	29	30	31
Medicine: Dose:																															
Overall relief:																															
Medicine: Dose:																															
Overall relief:																															
Medicine: Dose:																															
Overall relief:																															
Medicine: Dose:																															
Overall relief:																															
Medicine: Dose:																															
Overall relief:																															

PREVENTIVE MEDICINES
(Medicines to prevent headaches)

If you doctor has prescribed medicines for you, check (✓) off the day on the calendar every time you take a medicine.

Day of Month	1	2	3	4	5	6	7	8	9	10	11	12	13	14	15	16	17	18	19	20	21	22	23	24	25	26	27	28	29	30	31
Medicine: Dose:																															
Medicine: Dose:																															
Medicine: Dose:																															

PREVENTIVE LIFESTYLES

Day of Month	1	2	3	4	5	6	7	8	9	10	11	12	13	14	15	16	17	18	19	20	21	22	23	24	25	26	27	28	29	30	31
Exercise:																															
Relaxation performed																															

OVERALL SEVERITY FOR THIS MONTH   Circle one number

0	1	2	3	4	5	6	7	8	9	10
No problem										Almost unbearable

PHOTOCOPY MASTER **DIAGNOSIS**

Appendix B1 NECH headache calendar. Adapted with permission, The New England Center for Headache, Stanford, CT. ©1999 Glaxo Wellcome, Inc.

(continued)

MONITORING YOUR HEADACHES

You are about to use a very effective tool — the *Headache Calendar* — to help you and your providers determine how to best care for your headaches. By recording when you get your headaches, what medicines you took to relieve them, consider possible associations such as headache triggers including menses (when appropriate), patterns may be evident over time. These patterns will help direct needed changes in all forms of your treatments.

Before you use the *Headache Calendar*, review any instructions from your providers. Write the instructions below if they have not done so. Be sure to follow your practitioner's instructions exactly as prescribed or call 952-993-3432 for clarification.

Instructions from Your Doctor			
☐ **Acute Medicines** Take the following medicines to treat headache pain and related symptoms		☐ **Apnea/Sleep** _____ Regular to bed and regular to rise _____	
Medicine: _____ Dose: _____		☐ **Biofeedback/Relaxation Exercises and Time for Yourself** _____ Practice daily to near daily . Trial new technique: _____	
Medicine: _____ Dose: _____			
Medicine: _____ Dose: _____		☐ **Caffiene/Diet** _____ Restrict caffeine _____ _____ Eat 4-6 small portions daily _____ Restrict artificial sweeteners	
☐ **Preventive Medicines** Take the following medicines to help decrease how often you have headaches and the intensity of the headaches when they do occur.		☐ **Exercise** _____ Maintain current efforts _____ Increase by 15% every 1 to 2 weeks	
Medicine: _____ Dose: _____		☐ **Fluids:** _____ Maintain 8 -8ounces glasses water daily	
Medicine: _____ Dose: _____			
Medicine: _____ Dose: _____		☐ **Groups/ Social Connectedness/Other Special Instruction** _____	

HEADACHE TRIGGERS

Below are many things that provoke (trigger) headaches. (Circle) those that are believed to have provoked headache this month.

Headache Triggers

☐ **Hormones**
  1. Menses (period)
  2. Ovulation
  3. Hormone replacement therapy
  4. Oral contraceptives

☐ **Diet**
  5. Alcohol (especially beer and red wine)
  6. Chocolate
  7. Aged cheeses (Cheddar Gruyere, Brie, Camembert)
  8. Monosodium glutamate (MSG) — common in Chinese food
  9. Artificial sweeteners
  10. Caffeine
  11. Nuts
  12. Nitrates and nitrites (found in hot dogs, bologna, and other processed meats)
  13. Citrus fruits (grapefruit, oranges, lemons and their juices)
  14. Other: _____

☐ **Changes**
  15. Weather
  16. Seasons

  17. Travel (crossing a time zone)
  18. Altitude
  19. Schedule changes
  20. Sleeping patterns (too little, too much, or changes usual pattern)
  21. Diet
  22. Skipping meals

☐ **Sensory Stimuli**
  23. Strong lights
  24. Flickering lights
  25. Odors

☐ **Stress**
  26. Let-down periods (vacations, weekends, after a major event)
  27. Times of intense activity
  28. Loss (death, separation, divorce)
  29. Relationship difficulties
  30. Job stress, loss, or change
  31. Crisis
  32. Other: _____

PHOTOCOPY MASTER **DIAGNOSIS**

Appendix B1

To find out if you have menstrual migraines, copy the monthly calendar below so that you can track your periods, headaches, and possible triggers over a period of 3 to 6 months. Write in the days of the month in the smaller squared boxes.

Mark directly on the calendar the first and last day of your period, the day(s) you experience a headache or migraine; the pain intensity using a scale of 0 to 3 (0=No headache; 1=Mild; 2=Moderate; 3=Severe); and any possible triggers(s). See below for possible triggers and note the corresponding letter on the calendar if applicable. Bring the completed calendar(s) to your healthcare provider for a consultation.

Month/Year _____

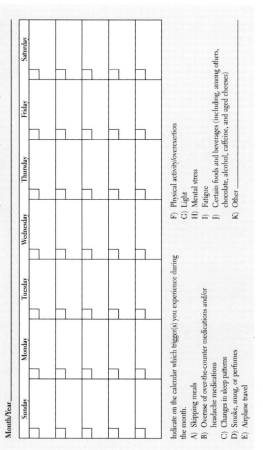

Sunday	Monday	Tuesday	Wednesday	Thursday	Friday	Saturday

Indicate on the calendar which trigger(s) you experience during the month.

A) Skipping meals
B) Overuse of over-the-counter medications and/or headache medications
C) Changes in sleep patterns
D) Smoke, smog, or perfumes
E) Airplane travel

F) Physical activity/overexertion
G) Light
H) Mental stress
I) Fatigue
J) Certain foods and beverages (including, among others, chocolate, alcohol, caffeine, and aged cheeses)
K) Other _____

Appendix B2 Sample headache calendar.

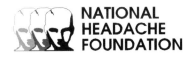

NATIONAL HEADACHE FOUNDATION

KEEPING A HEADACHE DIARY CAN HELP YOUR DOCTOR HELP YOU

NHF suggests answering the following questions to compile your headache history:

- When did you start having headaches?
- How often do they occur? At what time of day? During the week or on weekends? How long do they last?
- Where is the pain?
- Which word best describes it: throbbing, pounding, splitting, stabbing, blinding?
- Are your headaches associated with your menstrual cycle?
- What triggers your headache: certain foods, certain physical activities, bright light, strong odors, change in temperature or altitude, noise, smoke, stress, oversleeping?
- What symptoms do you experience prior to the headache?
- Does anyone else in your family suffer from headaches?
- Do you notice visual disturbances before or after your headaches?
- Do you suffer from more than one type of headache?

It is important to make an appointment with your doctor for the specific purpose of addressing your headache history rather than discussing headaches as part of a physician visit for other reasons. The National Headache Foundation also recommends keeping a diary to track the characteristics of your headaches. Patterns identified from your diary may help your doctor determine which type of headache you have and the most beneficial treatments.

For more information about headache causes and treatments, visit the NHF web site at *www.headaches.org* or call 888-NHF-5552.

Appendix B3 National Headache Foundation headache diary. Reprinted with permission, National Headache Foundation.

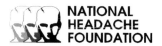

**NATIONAL
HEADACHE
FOUNDATION**

A headache diary consists of tracking the following information:

DATE	TIME (start/finish)	INTENSITY rate 1-10 (most severe being 10)	PRECEDING SYMPTOMS	TRIGGERS	MEDICATION (and dosage)	RELIEF (complete/moderate/none)

Appendix B3 For more information about headache causes and treatments, visit the NHF website at *www.headaches.org* or call 888-NHF-5552.

Appendix C

(VERSION 1.1)

This questionnaire was designed to help you describe and communicate the way you feel and what you cannot do because of headaches.

To complete, please circle one answer for each question.

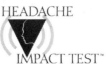

1 When you have headaches, how often is the pain severe?

| Never | Rarely | Sometimes | Very Often | Always |

2 How often do headaches limit your ability to do usual daily activities including household work, work, school, or social activities?

| Never | Rarely | Sometimes | Very Often | Always |

3 When you have a headache, how often do you wish you could lie down?

| Never | Rarely | Sometimes | Very Often | Always |

4 In the past 4 weeks, how often have you felt too tired to do work or daily activities because of your headaches?

| Never | Rarely | Sometimes | Very Often | Always |

5 In the past 4 weeks, how often have you felt fed up or irritated because of your headaches?

| Never | Rarely | Sometimes | Very Often | Always |

6 In the past 4 weeks, how often did headaches limit your ability to concentrate on work or daily activities?

| Never | Rarely | Sometimes | Very Often | Always |

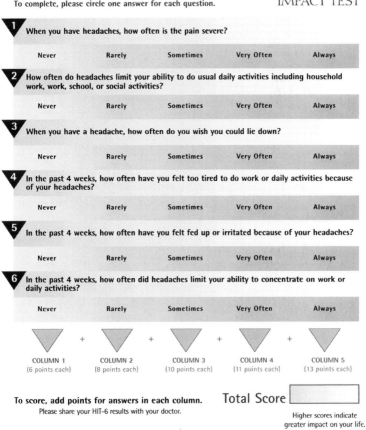

	+		+		+		+	
COLUMN 1		COLUMN 2		COLUMN 3		COLUMN 4		COLUMN 5
(6 points each)		(8 points each)		(10 points each)		(11 points each)		(13 points each)

To score, add points for answers in each column.
Please share your HIT-6 results with your doctor.

Total Score [   ]

Higher scores indicate greater impact on your life.

Score range is 36-78.

Appendix C1 HIT—Headache Impact Test. ©2001 QualityMetric, Inc. and GlaxoSmithKline Group of Companies. All rights reserved.

81

MIDAS QUESTIONNAIRE

This page contains the complete MIDAS Questionnaire, which can be used by physicians, pharmacists and patients. Questions 1 to 5 are used to calculate the MIDAS score. Questions A and B measure the frequency of the migraine and the severity of headache pain. They are not used to reach the MIDAS score, but provide extra information that physicians may find useful in making their treatment decisions.

INSTRUCTIONS: Please answer the following questions about ALL your headaches you have had over the last three months. Write your answer in the box next to each question. Write zero if you did not do the activity in the last 3 months. Please 'tab' through all five boxes to calculate your MIDAS score.

1 On how many days in the last 3 months did you miss work or school because of your headaches? ☐ days

2 How many days in the last 3 months was your productivity at work or school reduced by half or more because of your headaches? *(Do not include days you counted in question 1 where you missed work or school)* ☐ days

3 On how many days in the last 3 months did you not do household work because of your headaches? ☐ days

4 How many days in the last 3 months was your productivity in household work reduced by half or more because of your headaches? *(Do not include days you counted in question 3 where you did not do household work)* ☐ days

5 On how many days in the last three months did you miss family, social or leisure activities because of your headaches? ☐ days

Your rating: ☐ **TOTAL:** ☐ days

Appendix C2 MIDAS Questionnaire. ©1997 Innovative Medical Research.

A On how many days in the last 3 months did you have a headache? *(If a headache lasted more than 1 day, count each day)* ☐ days

B On a scale of 0-10, on average how painful were these headaches? *(Where 0 = no pain at all, and 10 = pain as bad as it can be)* ☐

Grade	Definition	Score
I	Minimal or infrequent disability	0-5
II	Mild or infrequent disability	6-10
III	Moderate disability	11-20
IV	Severe disability	21+

© Innovative Medical Research 1997

The MIDAS programme is sponsored by AstraZeneca

Appendix C2 *(continued)*

Appendix D

PATIENT HEALTH QUESTIONNAIRE (PHQ-9)

NAME: _____ DATE: _____

Over the *last 2 weeks,* how often have you been bothered by any of the following problems? *(use "✓" to indicate your answer)*	Not at all	Several days	More than half the days	Nearly every day
1. Little interest or pleasure in doing things	0	1	2	3
2. Feeling down, depressed, or hopeless	0	1	2	3
3. Trouble falling or staying asleep, or sleeping too much	0	1	2	3
4. Feeling tired or having little energy	0	1	2	3
5. Poor appetite or overeating	0	1	2	3
6. Feeling bad about yourself—or that you are a failure or have let yourself or your family down	0	1	2	3
7. Trouble concentrating on things, such as reading the newspaper or watching television	0	1	2	3
8. Moving or speaking so slowly that other people could have noticed. Or the opposite—being so fidgety or restless that you have been moving around a lot more than usual	0	1	2	3
9. Thoughts that you would be better off dead, or of hurting yourself in some way	0	1	2	3

add columns: _____ + _____ + _____

(Healthcare professional: For interpretation of TOTAL, please refer to accompanying scoring card.) **TOTAL:** _____

10. If you checked off *any* problems, how *difficult* have these problems made it for you to do your work, take care of things at home, or get along with other people?	**Not difficult at all** _____
	Somewhat difficult _____
	Very difficult _____
	Extremely difficult _____

Appendix D Patient Health Questionnaire (PHQ-9). ©1999 Pfizer Inc. All rights reserved. Reprinted with permission.

Appendix E

Headache Resource Information

Patient resources

American Council of Headache Education (ACHE)
    19 Mantua Road
    Mount Royal, NJ 08061
    (856) 423-0258
    (867) 423-0082 (fax)
    www.achenet.org

National Headache Foundation (NHF)
    820 N. Orleans, Ste 217
    Chicago, IL 60610-3132
    (888) NHF-5552
    www.headaches.org

National Menstrual Migraine Coalition
    www.headachesinwomen.org

Provider resources

American Headache Society (AHS)
    19 Mantua Road
    Mount Royal, NJ 08061
    www.ahsnet.org
    (856) 423-0043

National Headache Foundation
    820 N. Orleans, Ste 217
    Chicago, IL 60610-3132
    (888) NHF-5552
    www.headaches.org

National Menstrual Migraine Coalition
    www.headachesinwomen.org

Suggested reading for providers (journal articles)

Brandes JL. The influence of estrogen on migraine: A systematic review. *Journal of the American Medical Association.* 2006;295:1824–1830.

Calhoun A. Four hypotheses for understanding menstrual migraine. *The Female Patient.* 2004;29:38–43.

Hutchinson S. Menstrual migraine: The role of hormonal management. *The Female Patient.* 2007;32:54–58.

Loder E, et al. Women with migraine: Treatment opportunities and pitfalls. *Women's Health in Primary Care.* 2004;7:19–26.

Peterlin BL, Loder EW. Premenstrual headache: Diagnostic and pathophysiologic considerations. *Current Headache Reports.* 2006;5:193–199

Newman L, Silberstein SD. Prevention and management of menstrual migraine. *Current Headache Reports.* 2006;5:200–206.

Silberstein SD, Elkind AH, Schreiber C, et al. A randomized trial of frovatriptan for the intermittent prevention of menstrual migraine. *Neurology.* 2004;63:261–269.

Index